A
COURSE
IN
WEIGHT
LOSS

ALSO BY MARIANNE WILLIAMSON

*The Age of Miracles**

A Return to Love

A Woman's Worth

Illuminata

Emma & Mommy Talk to God

Healing the Soul of America

Illuminated Prayers

Enchanted Love

Everyday Grace

The Gift of Change

*Miracle Cards**

A Year of Daily Wisdom Perpetual Calendar*

*Available from Hay House

Please visit:

Hay House USA: **www.hayhouse.com**®
Hay House Australia: **www.hayhouse.com.au**
Hay House UK: **www.hayhouse.co.uk**
Hay House South Africa: **www.hayhouse.co.za**
Hay House India: **www.hayhouse.co.in**

A COURSE IN WEIGHT LOSS

21 SPIRITUAL LESSONS
FOR SURRENDERING
YOUR WEIGHT FOREVER

MARIANNE WILLIAMSON

HAY HOUSE

Australia • Canada • Hong Kong • India
South Africa • United Kingdom • United States

First published and distributed in the United Kingdom by:
Hay House UK Ltd, 292B Kensal Rd, London W10 5BE. Tel.: (44) 20 8962 1230;
Fax: (44) 20 8962 1239. www.hayhouse.co.uk

Published and distributed in the United States of America by:
Hay House, Inc., PO Box 5100, Carlsbad, CA 92018-5100. Tel.: (1) 760 431 7695
or (800) 654 5126; Fax: (1) 760 431 6948 or (800) 650 5115. www.hayhouse.com

Published and distributed in Australia by:
Hay House Australia Ltd, 18/36 Ralph St, Alexandria NSW 2015. Tel.: (61) 2 9669
4299; Fax: (61) 2 9669 4144. www.hayhouse.com.au

Published and distributed in the Republic of South Africa by:
Hay House SA (Pty), Ltd, PO Box 990, Witkoppen 2068. Tel./Fax: (27) 11 467
8904. www.hayhouse.co.za

Published and distributed in India by:
Hay House Publishers India, Muskaan Complex, Plot No.3, B-2, Vasant Kunj, New
Delhi – 110 070. Tel.: (91) 11 4176 1620; Fax: (91) 11 4176 1630. www.hayhouse.
co.in

Distributed in Canada by:
Raincoast, 9050 Shaughnessy St, Vancouver, BC V6P 6E5. Tel.: (1) 604 323 7100;
Fax: (1) 604 323 2600

A catalogue record for this book is available from the British Library.

ISBN 978-1-8485-0324-3

Printed and bound in Great Britain by TJ International, Padstow, Cornwall.

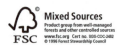

Mixed Sources
Product group from well-managed
forests and other controlled sources
FSC   www.fsc.org Cert no. SGS-COC-2482
© 1996 Forest Stewardship Council

For Oprah

This book began and ended as a communication between friends. Oprah Winfrey inspired the book, directed its course, and guided its vision. On a soul level definitely, and in many ways a literary one, this book was a collaborative effort. Every page is a reflection of my affection for and gratitude to her; my hope is that it brings comfort to her as she has brought comfort to so many.

To any reader who might feel that this book is a gift, please know that it was a gift from her.

~&~ CONTENTS ~&~

✣ FOREWORD ✣

In this wonderful and inspiring book by Marianne Williamson, she addresses the root causes not only of our weight, but also of our suffering.

For more than 30 years, my colleagues and I at the non-profit Preventive Medicine Research Institute have conducted a series of studies proving that when we address the underlying *causes* of a condition, our bodies often have a remarkable capacity to begin healing, and much more quickly than had once been thought possible. We've used high-tech, state-of-the-art measures to prove the power of these low-tech, low-cost, and ancient interventions.

Our research proved that the progression of even severe heart disease often can be reversed by making comprehensive lifestyle changes; so can early-stage prostate cancer as well as diabetes, high blood pressure, elevated cholesterol levels, arthritis, and depression. We published studies showing that when you change your lifestyle, you change your genes—turning on the genes that prevent disease and turning off the ones that promote heart disease, cancer, and other illnesses—and even increasing an enzyme that lengthens *telomeres* (the ends of our chromosomes that control aging), thereby enhancing longevity. And people lost an average of 24 pounds in the first year and kept off half that weight five years later.

However, if we only literally or figuratively *bypass* the underlying causes, then the same problem often recurs—we regain the lost weight, the bypassed coronary arteries clog up again, the medications have to be taken forever—or a new set of problems may occur, or there may be painful choices. When I lecture, I often show a slide of doctors busily mopping up the floor around an overflowing sink without also turning off the faucet.

The lifestyle choices we make each day in what we eat and in how we live are among the most important underlying causes of obesity and other chronic diseases. But there is an even deeper, root cause that powerfully affects our lifestyle choices, and that is the separation from who we really are—the misperception that we are separate and *only* separate. This is what Marianne describes so eloquently and intelligently in this book.

Information is important, but not usually sufficient, to motivate lasting changes in diet and lifestyle. If it were, we'd all be thin and healthy, as most people know which foods are healthy and unhealthy to eat. And no one would smoke. Everyone who smokes knows it's not good for them—the Surgeon General's warning is on every package of cigarettes, at least in this country. Yet one-third of Americans still smoke. Clearly, we need to work at a deeper level.

The real epidemic is not just obesity or heart disease or cancer; it's loneliness, depression, and isolation. If we address these deeper issues, then it becomes easier for people to make lasting changes in their behaviors.

In our studies, I spent a lot of time with the participants over a period of several years. We got to know each other very well, and a powerful trust emerged.

I asked them, "Teach me something. Why do you overeat? Smoke? Drink too much? Work too hard? Abuse substances? Watch too much television? Spend too much time on the Internet and video games? These behaviors seem so maladaptive to me."

They replied, "Dean, you just don't get it. These behaviors aren't maladaptive, they're *very* adaptive—because they help us get through the day. They numb our emotional pain."

Getting through the day becomes more important than living a long life when you're lonely, depressed, and isolated. As one patient told me, "I've got 20 friends in this pack of cigarettes. They're always there for me, and no one else is. You want to take away my 20 friends? What are you going to give me instead?"

Other patients take refuge in food. As someone once said to me, "When I feel lonely, I eat a lot of fat—it coats my nerves and numbs the pain. I can fill the void with food." There's a reason why fatty foods are often referred to as "comfort foods." We have many ways of numbing, bypassing, and distracting ourselves from pain.

Awareness is the first step in healing. Part of the benefit of pain is to get our attention, to help us make the connection between when we suffer and why, so we can make choices that are a lot more fun and healthful.

The experience of emotional pain and unhappiness can be a powerful catalyst for transforming not only behaviors like diet and exercise, but also for dealing with the deeper issues that really motivate us.

"Well, it may be hard to change, but I'm hurting so badly that I'm willing to try something new." At that point, properly guided, people are more willing to make lifestyle choices that are life-enhancing rather than those that are self-destructive.

Because the mechanisms that affect our health are so dynamic, when we work on a deeper level, we're likely to feel so much better, so quickly, that it reframes the reasons for change from fear of dying to joy of living.

What's sustainable are joy, pleasure, freedom, and love. Even more than being healthy and losing weight, most people want to feel free and in control.

Because of this, diets don't work. Diets are about what you *can't* have and what you *must* do. If you go *on* a diet, sooner or later you're likely to go *off* a diet. If you go *on* an exercise program, sooner or later you're likely to go *off* it.

And diets are often based on the fear that something really bad—like a heart attack, a stroke, or cancer—may happen to you otherwise. Efforts to try to motivate people to change their lifestyles based on fear don't work, because we don't want to believe that something really bad will ever happen to us, so we don't think about it.

Fear is not a sustainable motivator. Why? It's too scary. We all know we're going to die one day—the mortality rate is still 100 percent, one per person—but who wants to think about it? Even people who have had heart attacks usually change for only a few weeks before they go back to their old patterns of living and eating.

The language of behavioral change often has a moralistic quality to it that turns off a lot of people (like "cheating" on a diet). It's a small step from thinking of foods as "good" or "bad" to seeing yourself as a "good person" or a "bad person" if you eat these, and this creates downward spirals in a vicious cycle.

Also, the term "patient compliance" has a fascist, creepy quality to it, sounding like one person manipulating or bending his or her will to another. In the short run, I may be able to pressure you into changing your diet, but sooner or later (usually sooner), some part of you will rebel. (Remember, "Don't eat the apple" didn't work, and that was God talking. . . .)

And willpower is just another way of saying you're forcing yourself to do something, and pressuring yourself to do something is not sustainable. Again, what's sustainable are love, joy, pleasure, and freedom.

When we inevitably go off a diet, then we usually blame ourselves. Thus, humiliation, guilt, anger, and shame are inherent in most diet and lifestyle programs, and these are among the most toxic emotions.

Instead, with Marianne as our guide, we can go back to the root cause of our suffering: we've forgotten who we really are. *Health* comes from the root "to make whole." The word *yoga* derives from the Sanskrit word meaning "to yoke," to bring together. Science is helping to document the wisdom of ancient traditions.

Intimacy is healing. Trust is everything, because we can only be intimate to the degree we can make ourselves emotionally vulnerable. A fully committed relationship allows both people to feel complete trust in each other. Trust allows us to feel safe. When we feel safe, we can open our heart to the other person and be completely naked and vulnerable to him or her—physically, emotionally, and spiritually. When our heart is fully open and vulnerable, we can experience profound levels of intimacy that are healing, joyful, powerful, creative, and intensely ecstatic. We can surrender to each other out of strength and wisdom—not out of fear, weakness, and submission.

If that trust has been violated by physical, sexual, or emotional abuse—especially if it's by a parent or relative who is supposed to protect us—then intimacy can be dangerous and frightening. Overeating often becomes a way of protecting us from further abuse, but it also isolates us from the healing intimacy that we most want.

The values of community, compassion, forgiveness, altruism, and service are part of almost all religious and spiritual traditions as well as many secular ones—what the German philosopher Leibniz called "the perennial philosophy"—the common, eternal underpinnings of all religions once you get past the rituals and forms that are all too often used to divide rather than unify.

Altruism, compassion, and forgiveness may be healing for both the giver and the recipient because giving to others with an open heart helps heal the isolation and loneliness that separate us from each other. When we forgive others, it doesn't excuse their actions; it frees us from our own stress and suffering. These allow for deep levels of intimacy and community that are powerfully healing. When you meet hatred with love, and fear with hope, this transforms *you*, as well as those around you.

The ancient swamis and rabbis, monks and nuns, mullahs and maharishis, didn't use spiritual practices simply as powerful stress-management techniques, although they are. They are also powerful tools for transformation and transcendence, providing a direct experience of what it means to be happy and peaceful if we simply stop disturbing our natural state of inner peace.

These techniques do not *bring* peace and happiness; they simply help us to experience and rediscover the inner peace that is there already, once we stop disturbing it. As the ecumenical spiritual teacher Swami Satchidananda often said, "I'm not a Hindu; I'm an Un-do."

Prayer and meditation allow us to access our inner wisdom more intentionally. Have you ever awakened in the middle of the night and figured out the answer to a problem that had been troubling you? All spiritual traditions describe a "still, small voice within," a voice that speaks very clearly but very quietly. It's easily drowned out by the chatter and business of everyday life. For many people, the only time the mind is quiet enough to hear one's inner voice is when waking up in the middle of the night. Sometimes it says, "Listen up, pay attention. I have something important to tell you."

At the end of a meditation session—whether it's been one minute or one hour—my mind is much quieter and calmer, so I can hear the still, small voice within more clearly. I then ask myself, "What am I not paying attention to that I need to hear?" And then I wait, and listen.

Over time, I've learned to trust and recognize my inner voice. Everyone can. When we practice listening to our inner voice in quiet moments, we can learn to access it at the stressful times when we most need it.

If we pay attention to our inner wisdom, we can often recognize problems in their earlier stages when they are easier to rectify. As Oprah Winfrey once said, "Listen to the whisper before it becomes a scream."

Meditation, prayer, and other spiritual practices can provide the direct experience of the interconnectedness of life. On one level, we're all separate and apart from each other. You're you, and I'm me.

On another level, spiritual practices, taken deeply enough, allow us to experience that we are a part of something much larger that connects us, whatever name we give to that (even to give it a name is to limit what is a limitless experience). We are *a part of*, not just *apart from*, everyone and everything. We are That. In this context, love is not something we get; it's who we are.

When we can maintain that "double vision"—both the duality and the underlying unity—then we can enjoy life more fully and accomplish even more without so much suffering and stress, from a place of wholeness rather than lacking, from a feeling of interconnectedness rather than separateness and isolation. Our lives become manifestations of love, acts of love—the most powerful force in the universe.

And, by the way, you're likely to lose weight and keep it off, because lasting weight loss is a by-product of a deeper healing. This book brilliantly illuminates a path out of the darkness.

— **Dean Ornish, M.D.**, Founder and President, Preventive Medicine Research Institute; Clinical Professor of Medicine, University of California, San Francisco • **www.pmri.org**

ᴐ᷿᷾ᴐ INTRODUCTION ᴐ᷿᷾ᴐ

This book is a spiritual curriculum consisting of 21 lessons. It is separate from anything else you might do regarding diet or exercise. It is a retraining of your consciousness in the area of weight.

Perhaps you've made amazing efforts to lose weight in the past—employing everything from extraordinary diet plans to almost superhuman feats of exercise—yet have found yourself mysteriously unable to keep the weight off permanently. While you succeeded for a time in changing your behavior, you've not yet experienced the deep level of change necessary in order to truly solve the problem.

On your own you might have changed your conscious thinking, but you alone cannot change your subconscious. And unless your *subconscious* mind is enrolled in your weight-loss efforts, it will find a way to reconstitute the excess weight regardless of what you do.

Spirit alone has the power to positively and permanently reprogram both your conscious and subconscious mind. The holistic healing of any condition involves applying internal as well as external powers, and compulsive overeating is no different. This course is a lesson plan in aligning your thinking with the spiritual principles that will set you free.

The principles that guide these lessons are not difficult, but they are different from the way you might normally think. The principles are these:

1. Your body itself is completely neutral. It causes nothing; it is completely an effect, not a cause.

2. Neither poor diet nor lack of exercise are the *cause* of your excess weight. Mind is cause; body is effect. The cause of your excess weight is in your mind.

3. The cause of your excess weight is fear, which is a place in your mind where love is blocked.

4. Fear expresses itself as subconscious urges, which then express themselves as either excessive and/or unhealthy eating habits and/or resistance to proper exercise. The ultimate effect of this—that is, excess weight—will only be permanently and fundamentally healed when the fear itself is rooted out.

The purpose of this course is to root out your fear, and to replace it with an inestimable love.

It might seem odd to consider that fear is the source of your weight problem, and yet it is. As your mind is trained to let go of its fear, your body will let go of its excess pounds. For that shift in thinking from fear to love is a miracle: the reprogramming of your consciousness on a causal level, freeing the level of bodily effects to transform from dysfunction to healing. This course is not about your relationship with food; it is about your relationship with love. For love is your true healer. And miracles occur naturally in the presence of love.

Love is that which both created and sustains you. It's both your connection to your true reality and your alignment with the positive flow of the universe. Remembering this Divine truth—that love is who you are—is key to your healing, for your relationship to food is an area where your nervous system has lost the memory of its Divine intelligence. As you remember your own Divine truth, the cells of your body will remember theirs.

The body has a natural intelligence for creating and maintaining the perfect weight for you as long as the mind is aligned with its own perfection. Your perfect weight is coded into the natural patterns of your true self, as your perfect *everything* is coded into the patterns of your true self. The *real* you knows exactly how to inhabit your body in the healthiest, happiest way, and will do so automatically when you reestablish conscious connection with spiritual reality. By getting back to the truth of who you really are, you will get to a place where all your problems with weight have disappeared.

Reconnection to your spiritual reality is achieved through a force called here Divine Mind. It is a gift from God that will return you to your sanity, whenever you choose to call on it. Your compulsion is a place where, in your spiritual forgetfulness, you go temporarily insane if even for a moment—just long enough to open the bag of potato chips that's the trigger to your binge food mania. Lost in this forgetfulness, you become confused in your thinking and are unable to say "No" when something truly harmful to your well-being is posing as a supportive and loving friend. Divine Mind is the counterforce to this temporary insanity; when you are lost in moments of spiritual forgetfulness, it will remind you who you are.

The consciousness of the human race is dominated by fear, which has coalesced in your life in the form of a particular behavioral pattern: compulsive overeating. In doing this course, you will command the spirit of fear to depart.

The power of love is perfect, creative, self-organizing, healthy, self-healing, and abundant. The power of fear is insane, destructive, violent, disease producing, and lacking. It expresses itself as an impostor self, perverting your true nature and making you behave in a way that is opposite of who you truly are. It is spiritually immature to underestimate the power of either of these two forces. Both of them are active, and both of them have their eyes on you. One wishes you well, and the other wishes you dead.

When subconscious forces lead a person into chronic self-destructive behavior over which their conscious mind has little or no control, this is called an addiction. Addiction is a system of self-generated behavior over which a merely self-generated psychological response system holds no sway. Addiction is when you can't stop. When some craziness takes over and you do or don't do whatever it is you do that blows it every time, ruins everything, snatches happiness from your hands, and leaves you desperate at what your life has become. It's life when lived at the behest of a wicked witch who seems to have taken over your brain and now uses it as her control room, directing you to do the most self-destructive things and then cackling with amusement as you lie writhing on the ground in misery right afterward.

Whether or not you are a food addict is something only you can say. Every food addict is a compulsive overeater, but not every compulsive eater is an addict. The principles in this course apply to both.

The love that will free you is a love that comes from *beyond* your mortal mind. It is a Divine intercession from a thought system beyond our own. Placing your problems in the hands of God, the situation it represents will be re-created. That which is imperfect will then become perfect.

Intellectually understanding your body, your mind-body connection, the physiology of exercise, or the realities of food metabolism mean little if you are addicted. In the words of Sigmund Freud, "Intelligence will be used in the service of the neurosis." The fact that you yourself have anything figured out makes little or no difference to any of this. No matter how smart you are, or how much "work you've done on yourself," you alone cannot outsmart the psychic force of compulsion and addiction. If you could, you would have done so by now. For this problem, entrenched and pernicious as it is, you need spiritual forces to help you. For this, you need God.

This course is not about food but about spirituality—the quest for a power that is greater than your own. It is not about your addiction, but about a force that is more powerful than your addiction. Our purpose is not to analyze your darkness but to turn on a light that, having been trapped within you, is now ready to blaze forth.

The spirit of fear is love inverted, or your own mental power turned against yourself. Have you ever found yourself saying something that you knew in your heart to be the opposite of how you really felt? In a moment of self-hate, your mind became so twisted as to convince you that you are acting out of self-love. "I'm eating all these cookies to *comfort myself.*" "I'm eating all this bread because it *nourishes me emotionally.*" It is not just your mind but also your body that can go insane. Compulsion and addiction render the life-sustaining proclivities of both mind and body temporarily inoperative. This is not a war that reason can win.

So ask yourself this question: *Are you willing, if even for a moment, to consider the possibility that God can outwit your insanity?* If you feel that on your own you simply cannot stop waging this war against yourself—a war that if unabated could eventually kill you—then allow yourself to surrender to a fervent hope and to feel, if even for a moment, that the help you've prayed for has finally arrived.

You would not be reading this course if you had not already come to this place. Sometimes we need to admit the darkness within us, and at other times we need to admit the light. At the deepest level, it is not your food obsession that you most need to admit to yourself. At the deepest level, it is the memory of your Divine light that you most need to admit to yourself . . . the light of God that lives within you as the gift that it is: the solution to every problem, even this one.

Dear God,
Please free me
from false appetites
and take away my pain.
Take from me my compulsive self,
and show me who I am.
Dear God,
Please give me a new beginning.
Unchain my heart
so I might live
a freer life at last.
Amen

~❧ EMBARKING ❧~ ON THE JOURNEY

You are about to embark upon a specific journey, and as with everything else in your life, you have two choices: you can play it shallow or you can play it deep.

The overeater has a delusional relationship with food, imbuing it with power it doesn't actually possess. Perhaps you've subscribed to the magical belief that eating affords you comfort and strength, even when you are eating food (or an amount of food) that in fact can only hurt you. The overeater forms an idolatrous relationship with food in which powers that belong only to God have been ascribed to something else.

Begin by simply seeing this.

Spiritual growth is a fascinating process when you allow it to be. It is an inner journey from one insight to another, in which helpful realizations fall into place as you are ready to receive them. Twisted thoughts become untwisted once you see them for what they are. Your journey from blindness to spiritual vision precedes your journey from dysfunctional eating to a healthy and wholesome relationship to food; in fact, it is a necessary prerequisite for it. As you understand more deeply the roots of your weakness, you lay the foundation for the cultivation of new strengths.

The first realization on your journey to freedom is that you have come to believe a lie. Then, through the strength of your belief in this lie, you have actually made it seem true for you. The lie is that food that is actually bad for you has the power to comfort, nurture, and sustain you. Your task is to correct the lie.

The line from the end of the Lord's Prayer, "For Thine is the kingdom, the power, and the glory," means "Only God has the power to comfort, nurture, and sustain me." That line is not an entreaty but an affirmation, which when said prayerfully has the power to penetrate the deepest regions of your subconscious mind. You are realizing that food cannot nurture you emotionally, and that God, and only God, can.

In giving all power to Spirit, you realign the energies of your subconscious mind; you thus beckon every aspect of yourself—including your body—back to Divine right order. Your body is meant to be a reflection of your spirit, and both your thoughts and your cells will respond to a reminder of their Divine perfection.

The goal of this course is to remind your body of its perfection by reminding your mind of its perfection. By resetting one, you reset the other.

This course is cumulative. Every day you will be given a lesson, and while the content of that lesson is to be focused on for a particular day, its energy should be allowed to live continuously within your psyche as the days unfold. Compulsive eating involves two things: compulsion and food. You will not end your compulsive eating by substituting another compulsive practice. Therefore, this is not a course to race through, but rather a process to relax into.

These lessons are not meant to cause you consternation or feelings of guilt. They can neither be passed nor failed; *you* can neither be passed nor failed. Simply allow yourself to fall into them as into a gentle place, where you are equally loved whether you do the lesson "right" on any given day or you fall short. The only way you can "fail" a lesson is if you punish yourself for failing. This course is a journey, and as with any serious journey of self-discovery, there are days when we detour into darkness as we make our way toward light.

In moments that are difficult—perhaps you'll read something inspiring in one of the lessons and close your eyes for a beautiful and peaceful time of meditation, but then find yourself an hour later finishing a whole bag of potato chips!—know that the problem is not the potato chips, but rather the fear that has been aroused in the presence of love.

It has been said that love brings up everything unlike itself, and sometimes just when we feel we are moving toward a solution, the problem jumps up again and grabs us by the throat. That is natural. It is part of the process. Do not despair.

In such a situation, simply take a deep breath, acknowledge yourself for your efforts, and forgive yourself for the detour. Know that the patterns of light you are establishing now will in time cancel out all darkness. Know that the greatest successes are often arrived at two steps forward and then a step or two back. And know that skinny people eat too many potato chips sometimes, too.

These lessons are simple, but their potential to heal you is profound. The reason the lessons are gentle is because your overeating is not. Only the power of love can overcome the power of hate, and make no mistake about it: your unhealthy eating is an act of self-hate. Overeating is a form of violence, and one of the mechanisms you are now dismantling is your habit of taking up the sword against yourself—whether the sword be knife or fork.

Begin with a commitment to be kind to yourself. Over-eating is an emotionally violent act, and scolding yourself for having done it is just inflicting further violence. At some point you'll act out those feelings, and it's a pretty good bet you'll lean on your fallback position of overeating as your favorite way to express self-hate. Not only that, but the over-eating would then also be a perfect way to comfort yourself while feeling all that guilt.

Is the insanity becoming clear enough yet? And does it not follow that it would take a miracle to dismantle such a weird and twisted set of thoughts and emotions? At a certain point, you come to admit a truth that you previously resisted: you don't have the human capacity to fix this problem.

Yet that's not the end. It's only the beginning. For in realizing that you can't heal yourself, you begin to consider Who can.

These lessons are not just something you are going to read; doing this course requires your active participation. Occasionally you'll be asked to procure an item or two or to do an activity, and often you'll be asked to write things down. There are pages at the end of the book for this pur-pose, or you may wish to use a separate journal. Writing will be very useful to you throughout the course, as it will help you integrate the lessons more fully.

With that, let's begin our journey.

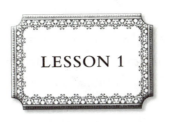

TEAR DOWN THE WALL

I was never a food addict, but for years I was a compulsive overeater. Diets did not work. I would starve myself, then binge, starve myself, then binge, in a constant cycle of self-abnegation and self-indulgence. I hated many things about the situation, but what was worse than anything else was how much I thought about food. I was obsessed with it. Thoughts of eating hardly ever left my mind.

And then they did, in a miraculous way. When I began studying *A Course in Miracles,* I wasn't consciously thinking of my weight as an area where I wanted a miracle. But one day I looked down and couldn't believe what I saw, on the scale or on my body. Weight had simply dropped off, and I realized why. The weight had merely been a physical manifestation of my need to keep others at bay. I feared other people and had built a wall to protect myself. Practicing the *Course,* I'd learned to extend my hand across the wall. I'd learned ways to replace fear with love. I'd asked God to enter my life and make all things right. And the wall had disappeared.

Your first lesson focuses on the following visualization: the image of excess weight as a brick wall you are carrying around. This wall has been built by your subconscious mind; its purpose is to separate you from other people and from life itself. Your fear has built the wall, and love will tear it down.

Looking closely, you see that every brick has something written on it:

Shame

Anger

Fear

Unforgiveness

Judgment

Disdain

Excess responsibility

Pressure

Exhaustion

Burden

Stress

Heartbreak

Injustice

Protection

Pride

Selfishness

Jealousy

Greed

Laziness

Separation

Dishonesty

Arrogance

Inferiority

Embarrassment

Self-abnegation

Now allow yourself to read this list again, very slowly. With every word, ask yourself whether or not it represents a thought, an emotional reality, or a character defect that pertains to you. Know that the vast majority of people, were they to be honest with themselves, would say "Yes." (You might even add a few words of your own to the list.) And with every word, move slowly into your heart and allow yourself to identify the situations or circumstances in your life that this word connects to.

The weight you are seeking to let go of was added to your consciousness before it was added to your body. Your body is merely a screen onto which is projected the nature of your thoughts. When the weight is gone from your consciousness, it will be gone from your physical experience. In asking God to remove the cause, you automatically remove the effect.

The weight on your mind, and thus on your body, is the weight of your own emotional shadows that have not yet had a light shone on them, whether they be unprocessed feelings, negative thoughts, or fear-based attitudes and personality traits. They are no different from the shadows that other people have.

What is unique to your situation is that for whatever reason, these thoughts or feelings have become frozen within you and are not being processed properly. Instead of your getting sad, let's say—going through the sadness and then moving to the other side of it—your sadness is likely, for various reasons, to stay stuck within your mind. And then it gets stuck within your body. You are failing to assimilate an experience and let it go. Emotionally and mentally, as well as physically, our systems must process waste.

Painful experiences are not meant to linger. They are meant to teach us what they need to teach us, and then dissolve into the realm of soft-focus memory. Even bitterness in our past can transform into peaceful acceptance. With your system of psychological-waste removal on the blink, however, you've subconsciously tried to get rid of these thoughts and feelings by eating them. *If I can't process my sadness, perhaps I can eat my sadness. If I can't process my anger, perhaps I can eat my anger.*

In the absence of an exit valve for what could be seen as your psychological sewage, your unprocessed thoughts and feelings have embedded themselves in your flesh—*literally*. They are the materialization of dense, unprocessed energy that had nowhere else to go. You are carrying your burdens around—not only with you but on you. This course is a way to release them to God.

It's not as though other people don't have unprocessed emotions; we all do. In some of us, unprocessed pain expresses itself through taking drugs or drinking; in others, through emotional outbursts; in still others, through promiscuous sex, and so forth. The form of dysfunction is not particularly relevant; what matters is that we address the unprocessed suffering behind it.

In order for your healing to be real and deep, you must be willing to be real and deep with the issues you address here. No one else needs to know what is revealed to you, unless you choose to share the information with a trusted friend. This journey is a sacred one, in which you travel with God through the secrets of your heart.

With this lesson, you'll begin to tear down the wall.

There are only two categories of thoughts—those of love and those of fear—and the only way to transcend fear is to replace it with love. As you identify fear thoughts and then surrender them to Divine Mind, love emerges naturally. When thoughts that lead you to overeat are surrendered, then those that lead you to wholesome eating come forth to take their place.

The unprocessed fear will then leave your system, in time taking with it the pounds of flesh it has produced. In bringing it into your conscious mind and surrendering it to God, your fear and then your excess weight will be transmuted and removed.

In the past, you may simply have ignored or suppressed the thoughts, feelings, and memories that caused you pain. By doing so, however, you stopped a natural process by which such thoughts and feelings could be transformed. The pain has been pushed into your flesh. Now you are remembering that you can make another choice: you can look at your pain, and then release it to One in Whose hands it will dissolve forever.

It is not enough to merely identify your pain; you must then surrender it for healing. Saying, for instance, "I am so embarrassed about this or that situation," is not of itself a healing. To say, "Dear God, I am so embarrassed about that situation. I place everything that happened and all my feelings about it in Your hands. Please help me see it differently." *That* is a healing.

What is placed on the altar is then altered; as you surrender a situation, your thoughts about it are changed. Divine Mind comes into your worldly thoughts from a thought system beyond your own, authorized to return you to grace and sanity. You can think of this as a Divine intercession; this course is a lesson plan in miraculous thinking as applied to your efforts to lose weight. Divine Mind will remove the wall that surrounds you when you look at each brick, own your thoughts and feelings that imbue that brick with such addictive force, and then place it in His hands. Give to Him what you do not want, and what you do not want will disappear.

By recognizing what constitutes the wall around you, you will begin the process of dismantling it.

Return now to the words listed at the beginning of the chapter, which represent the bricks in your wall. For each word, write down in your journal what is true for you. Do not rush through this process. Be as detailed and complete as you can, feeling free to go back to certain words after you've already moved on to others. Allow yourself to look and to feel, and you will ultimately understand. This is a meaningful opportunity to see your light, by being courageous enough to look at your darkness.

Shame: *I am ashamed of* _____.
Perhaps you acted foolishly, and cringe to think that other people still remember. . . .
Do not go unconscious. Write it all out.

Anger: *I am angry at* _____.
Perhaps you feel unfairly treated, and have not released all your anger at the meanness of others. Or perhaps you have not forgiven yourself for self-sabotaging behavior in the past that affects your life now. . . .
Do not go unconscious. Write it all out.

Fear: *I am afraid of* _____.
Perhaps you carry a secret fear of loss, of tragedy, and have not yet learned to release it to God. . . .
Do not go unconscious. Write it all out.

Unforgiveness: *I haven't forgiven* _____ *for* _____.
Perhaps there is someone who betrayed your heart and you have not been able to forgive him or her yet. . . .
Do not go unconscious. Write it all out.

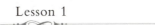
Judgment: *I judge* _____ *for* _____

_____.

Perhaps you think that others are behaving in ways they shouldn't, and you think and/or speak of them in negative terms. . . .

Do not go unconscious. Write it all out.

Disdain: *I feel disdain for* _____.

Perhaps there are those who disagree with you, and you hold contempt for their beliefs and actions. . . .

Do not go unconscious. Write it all out.

Excess responsibility: *I am responsible for* _____

_____.

Perhaps you carry the burden of thinking you're responsible for things that are out of your control. . . .

Do not go unconscious. Write it all out.

Pressure: *I feel so pressured about* _____.

Perhaps you feel that at home, at work, as a lover, as a friend, as an employee, or as a parent, you're carrying more pressure than you can stand. . . .

Do not go unconscious. Write it all out.

Exhaustion: *I am exhausted because* _____.

Perhaps you feel physically, mentally, and emotionally so tired that you can hardly stand to awaken some days. . . .

Do not go unconscious. Write it all out.

Burden: *I am burdened by* _____.

Perhaps you are carrying a pain in your heart that lies heavy upon you and weighs you down. . . .

Do not go unconscious. Write it all out.

Stress: I am stressed by _____.

Perhaps the bills you owe, the responsibilities you carry, the needs of your family, the demands of work, and so forth are a constant source of stress. . . .

Do not go unconscious. Write it all out.

Heartbreak: My heart is heavy because _____ _____.

Perhaps someone you love is ill, or has left you, or has died. . . .

Do not go unconscious. Write it all out.

Injustice: It isn't fair that I _____.

Perhaps you were overlooked, or dissed, or thrown under the bus, or not treated fairly. Or perhaps you cannot stand the injustice that is perpetrated against others. . . .

Do not go unconscious. Write it all out.

Protection: I feel I need protection from _____ _____.

Perhaps you feel there is a person or a condition that is a threat to your well-being, that frightens you. . . .

Do not go unconscious. Write it all out.

Pride: I am prideful when _____.

Perhaps you lack humility when dealing with others, failing to listen to them deeply or to admit when you've made a mistake. . . .

Do not go unconscious. Write it all out.

Selfishness: I am selfish when _____.

Perhaps you grab for what you want in life without thinking of the needs of others. . . .

Do not go unconscious. Write it all out.

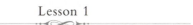
Jealousy: I get jealous when _____.

Perhaps you tear others down when you fear their success, not having learned that blessing others and what they have is a way of manifesting the same abundance in your own life. . . .

Do not go unconscious. Write it all out.

Greed: I get greedy when _____.

Perhaps you accumulate more than you need in life, giving no deference to moderation, balance, or the needs of others. . . .

Do not go unconscious. Write it all out.

Laziness: I am lazy when _____.

Perhaps you fail to take responsibility for generating energy in a positive, vital, and productive way. . . .

Do not go unconscious. Write it all out.

Separation: I feel separate from _____.

Perhaps there is a friend or family member or organization or community from which you've been disconnected, leaving a pain in your heart. . . .

Do not go unconscious. Write it all out.

Dishonesty: I don't feel that I can be honest about _____
_____.

Perhaps you carry a secret, something you don't feel you can safely tell anyone. Perhaps it's a guilty secret, or something that you simply fear others would judge you for. . . .

Do not go unconscious. Write it all out.

Arrogance: I am better than _____.

Perhaps you think you are smarter, better, more qualified, or more worthy than someone else . . . perhaps you feel your sensitivity makes you superior. . . .

Do not go unconscious. Write it all out.

Inferiority: I feel not as good as _____.
Perhaps you feel that others are smarter, better, more qualified, or more worthy than you . . . perhaps you feel that your weight makes you inferior. . . .
Do not go unconscious. Write it all out.

Embarrassment: I feel embarrassed because _____
_____.
Perhaps you have fallen down in some way in front of others . . . perhaps your issues with weight have increased this embarrassment . . . perhaps your spouse or children are embarrassed by your appearance. . . .
Do not go unconscious. Write it all out.

Self-abnegation: I have built this wall so that others won't hate me for being beautiful and successful and seeming to have it all _____.
Perhaps you have subconsciously chosen excess weight as a bargaining chip to win the approval of others, as though if you still have one big thing you suffer from, then you're not so glorious as to offend them. . . .
Do not go unconscious. Write it all out.

Reflection and Prayer

Closing your eyes, see yourself standing in a golden light.
See all the flesh you think of as excess weight as a brick wall that you carry around. Looking closely at the wall, see that it is made up of your own suffering and pain.
Now ask God to walk up to the wall with you. Together, the two of you begin to take down each brick, one by one, and ultimately dismantle the wall. Explain to Him what each brick means to you, then watch how whenever He touches a brick, it crumbles.

Do not rush away from this vision; rather, hold it for as long as you can. Spirit will illumine your understanding and give you the permission to feel the pain that you've denied for so long. And the pain will begin to leave. . . .

Dear God,
Please remove the wall that I have built around me.
I have built it so strong,
dear God,
that I cannot tear it down.
I surrender to You
every thought of separation,
every feeling of fear,
every unforgiving thought.
Please, dear God,
take this burden
from me forever.
Amen

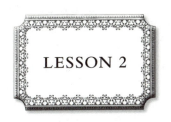

THIN YOU, MEET NOT-THIN YOU

Today's lesson involves your getting to know, and to love, the part of you that overeats.

There are parts of you the way there are parts of the color blue. There is pastel blue, which is blue mixed with white. There is dark blue, which is blue mixed with black. There is purplish blue, which is blue mixed with red. All of them are blue, yet they are different hues of one color. The one thing they have in common is blue itself.

So it is with you. Like everyone, you are a multidimensional being. There are many facets to you, all living together within your psyche. These differing "selves" are part of a mosaic that makes up the entirety of who you are.

There is the you in which your basic identity is mixed with a healed heart and high self-esteem; that's you when you're happy, healthy, and successful. And then there is the you in which your basic identity is mixed with trauma and low self-worth; that's you when you're neurotic, compulsive, addictive, and so forth. What all these parts of you have in common is *you*, manifesting in many different ways

31

depending on a variety of factors and experiences throughout your life.

You might express beautifully, serenely, and lovingly in
one aspect of your personality; yet meanly, frantically, and
fearfully in another. Everyone is a mix of characteristics—
few people are all perfect, or all imperfect. Yet those places
where you're imperfect are not where you're bad; they're
simply where you're wounded. And what has wounded you,
in one way or another, is fear itself.

For the overeater, food is an area where a spirit of fear
has infected the nervous system in a particular area, like a
virus in a bio-computer mixing all the settings and causing a malfunction. In other areas of your life, you might be
competent and happy and successful. But when it comes
to eating—a fundamental ingredient of a healthy life—it's
as though wires have gotten crossed in your brain. What is
unhealthy can seem good; what is good can seem boring.
When the brain reports something as comforting that in
fact is actually harmful, or the physical appetites crave what
the body knows it doesn't want, this confusion of signals is
so deep that the rational mind alone cannot fix it.

Our lesson today involves the miraculous transformation
of a certain part of you—not through denial but through
embrace. Your lesson today involves learning to love the
not-thin you, for she is nothing other than a product of fear;
and fear, being the absence of love, is a call for love. A part
of you that is a manifestation of fear cannot be transformed
by fear. Miracles arise only in the spirit of love. The way to
transform a malfunction is to treat it functionally. And your
only true function is love.

When you have surrendered yourself to the spirit of love,
when you have allowed Divine Mind to enter the inner-
most chambers of your heart, when you have opened your
eyes to the darkness within you and come at last upon the

light, then fear will dissolve. And as the spirit of fear dissolves within your consciousness, love will heal you, body and soul.

You're *you*, whether you're eating wisely or eating excessively. But when you're eating wisely, you're expressing love for yourself. When you're eating excessively, you're expressing fear. Love dissolves fear the way light dissolves darkness. Fat cells will dissolve *permanently* when they are dissolved through the power of love.

Any reaction to your not-thin self that is based on fear will only keep your excess weight in place. If the miracle you are seeking is the removal of excess weight, then learning to love all aspects of yourself—*even her*—is your liberation.

As counterintuitive as it sounds, it is your learning to love Not-Thin You that will cause this aspect of yourself to disappear. She didn't ask to be here; she isn't comfortable here; she was summoned up, and summoned up by *you*. As you make her your ally rather than your enemy, she will disappear into the light of your true being. She is quite literally a manifestation of a ghost, a mere twisted thought given form by your subconscious mind. But before love, or ultimate reality, *all that is nothing.*

Nothing. . . ? How can that be? How can this problem be *nothing?* And herein lies the secret of miracles: that fear is as nothing before the power of God. Love is ultimately real because it is Divine; fear is ultimately unreal because it is not. In the presence of God's love, illusions disappear.

The physical eye perceives only physical reality, and physical reality itself is but a dream of the mortal mind. Your spiritual eye extends your perception to the spiritual reality beyond the material world. And what you see beyond this world, you have the power to draw into it. As you learn to *see* your perfect self—knowing it is there because it exists in the mind of God—your mortal world will come to reflect it. Developing your spiritual eye is the key to your transformation, for in filling your eye with light, darkness disappears.

Your problem may be manifest on the level of the body, but it will be solved on the level of spirit. Learning to think about your problem in spiritual terms will lead you to its solution, because it will release the power of your spirit to work on your behalf. As you learn to align your thinking with spiritual truth, then you will enter a dimension where nothing but love can touch you. Fear will be rendered inoperative, and your compulsion will be gone.

As powerful as your compulsion to overeat might be, it is powerless before the power of the Divine. The energies and experiences that led to the development of your dysfunctional relationship with food *are as nothing before the will of God*. As you claim the totality of who you really are, who you really aren't will simply melt away.

Today's lesson involves healing the relationship between the part of you that eats wisely, and the part of you that eats dysfunctionally. They are not two separate beings, but rather two aspects of one mind. They cannot be separated by force, but only by love.

These two facets of you manifest as Thin You and Not-Thin You. They are energetically as well as physically different. Thin You is beautiful in a 21st-century kind of way, and therefore your conscious mind wants to inhabit her. Not-Thin You is beautiful as well, however, in an ancient kind of way. There is nothing inherently or objectively unattractive about your Not-Thin self, and that is important to realize. She is not ugly; she is simply you with a coat on, and you would prefer to take it off.

To judge an aspect of yourself as ugly is to abuse yourself, and then you might respond to your hurt by . . . let's say . . . grabbing something to eat. Obviously, this conflict keeps

34

you in a chronic pattern of self-hate and self-sabotage, kept under control at times but never fully healed. Your desire is to take off your coat, not pile on another one.

The purpose of this lesson is to support you in reconciling your relationship with Not-Thin You. She is not your enemy; she is an unintegrated part of yourself. She is an aspect of you that is demanding to be seen and heard. It is only in learning to love her that you'll gain the power to calm her down. "I thought if I put this coat on, I'd be big enough to get your attention." And you have to admit, she *has* gotten your attention.

You are understandably ambivalent about developing a conscious relationship with Not-Thin You, as you fear that in honoring her, you will be granting her permission to stay. Your natural inclination might be to think that in embracing her, you will fortify her presence—how could it be helpful to go *toward* that which one is hoping will go away? Yet only by embracing her, will you compel her to leave.

It does feel odd that we should honor a part of ourselves that we do not want, but Not-Thin You will not go away until she is listened to. You don't want her physical manifestation, but you *do* want a message that she carries with her. She is simply waiting for you to receive it and she can go. Once she is accepted as the part of you that you have made a habit of disowning, she will dissolve into the nothingness from whence she came. She will not leave until you love yourself. All of yourself. Including her. Period.

Does a parent love a troubled child less than the untroubled child? In accepting Not-Thin You, you are not accepting her weight; you are simply accepting *her*. And in accepting her, you are accepting the totality of yourself. As an aspect of yourself, Not-Thin You longs for nothing more than to be congruent with every other part of you. When she is accepted for who she is, she will become who she *truly* is.

She will merge into the gestalt of your highest-functioning self, which, among other things, inhabits your physical body at its perfect weight.

Part of your inner conflict is that while your conscious mind feels a level of disdain for Not-Thin You, your subconscious mind feels quite at home with her. On a subconscious level, you might feel more comfortable within a larger body. There is something you *allow* yourself when you are manifesting as Not-Thin You. At times she feels more like the "real" you. Consciously, you feel like Thin You is the *real* you, while Not-Thin You is the imposter; but *subconsciously*, you feel like Not-Thin You is the real you, and *Thin You* is the imposter.

The experience everyone yearns for is love, and you have come to experience eating as an act of self-love, even when you are eating unwisely. Even when you overeat—an act you know better than to think of as *actual* self-love, given that it is inherently self-destructive—you experience yourself as emotionally nourished, even if it's just for a moment. A subconscious effort at self-love turns into an act of self-hate. As you transform—as you learn to be fed love by love itself—you will stop looking to food for what food cannot feed you.

You will learn a new set of habits. When you are about to put something into your mouth that you know is not healthy, either in quantity or quality, you will love yourself too much to continue: you will stop, take a deep breath, and feel love enter your mouth instead. Love will travel down through your throat and enter every cell of your being, healing it and returning it to Divine right order. This process will actually shrink your stomach by building and repairing your system of physical appetites.

Today you'll begin a new relationship with a part of yourself you've kept out of your heart. For in keeping her *out* of your heart, you've kept her *on* your body. Until you do this, you will continue with what years of habit have taught you to do with conflict: reach for food as someone else might reach for a drink or a drug.

Your pain is exacerbated by the fact that other addictions can be kept secret, at least for a length of time. Yours cannot, which increases your self-loathing, which increases your conflict, which increases your eating, which increases your weight, which increases your suffering . . . until God steps in.

This lesson establishes an honorable and honoring connection with a particular aspect of yourself, Not-Thin You, based not on disgust but on appreciation. As you build this relationship, reintegrating an aspect of yourself that clearly will not be denied anyway, then you will regain your authority as ruler of yourself. What you do not love, you do not understand. And with what you do not understand, you cannot negotiate.

Learning to love Not-Thin You, bringing her back into the circle of your compassion, you will gain dominion over your life. Love will harmonize your internal kingdom. This aspect of you only appears as large because she feels you are not looking at her, and she is trying to tell you something. She will not go away until she is accepted for who she is. Once she does feel accepted back into your heart, she will automatically respond to your desire that she manifest differently.

Metaphysically, this is called *shape-shifting*. Your goal is not to *push her out*, but to *let her in*. At that point, having been psychically reintegrated into your spirit, she will have no further need to manifest physically at all.

Reflection and Prayer

If you're angry at someone, then it's hard to just say, "I love you, I love you," and that's it, all is forgiven. Sometimes you have to express your upset with that person before you can forgive him or her. How can you come to love Not-Thin You when somewhere in your heart you probably hate her?

In *A Course in Miracles,* it's said that miracles are born of total communication given and received. There's no point pretending that it's *easy* to love Not-Thin You, given how much pain, shame, fatigue, and self-hatred she's caused you. You might intellectually understand that she's a manifestation of your thoughts, but that doesn't of itself make her go away.

What you're going to do now is initiate a dialogue with Not-Thin You based on honesty and transparency. A part of you has dissociated from another part of you. That dissociation has led to a profound dysfunction, as one part of you has acted against the interests of the other. It's time to integrate the different parts of yourself, in order to end the battle that's been raging within you. It's time to write a couple of letters. It's time for peace talks.

Having asked Divine Mind to guide your process, settle into a relaxed space. Now with your inner eye, see Not-Thin You standing before you. Begin a dialogue with her. Open your heart and allow a process of communication between these two aspects of yourself to unfold.

Your work here is to share your truth . . . to tell Not-Thin You how you really feel . . . how you feel she has ruined your happiness . . . how much you hate her even, if indeed you do. Include the "I hate you, get out of my life" type of things. This letter is for no one's eyes but yours alone, but it is an important thing to write. You are not writing these things in order to attack Not-Thin You, but simply to communicate with her . . . to begin a dialogue that allows you to surrender thoughts that are already there, but that if unexplored remain as toxins in your system.

Although the point is not to hate Not-Thin You, you cannot get to love without first acknowledging what stands before it. Once you have told your truth to Not-Thin You and then allowed her to respond, you will learn a very important truth: she does not stand before you craving food; she stands before you craving love.

As with the writing you did regarding the bricks in the wall, neither rush through this process nor leave anything out. Tell the truth, the whole truth, and nothing but the truth.

Below is a letter expressing how a woman named Beatrice communicated to her not-thin self:

Dear Fat Ass,

I know your lumps and bumps are merely a navigational reminder of where you have been, of the things that were out of your control and happened early on. When Bad Things Happen to Little Girls. All of that. The Story. The Events. But now, you are the Event. He no longer has control over what happens to you, Fatty. The double-cheese pizza and nachos are no longer where it's at. You are here. You can celebrate your fierceness that was born with me, Skinny You, long ago, when you stood up and spit in his face. With push-ups and cute bras, that miracle of a miniskirt that has been hanging in your closet since 1992, with bike rides and mountain climbing and long swims in the sea. Not with the hourly walk to the fridge to see what might make Fat You feel better in the middle of the night—he's not coming for you anymore. You made sure of it years ago. We did it together.

Put down the fork and pick up the fight!

Put the cheeseburger down and go for a hike in beautiful Hollywood! Walk the streets and listen to your music, let Bob Dylan tell you how it is, listen to Bono and let those hips subside! I'm here! I'm waiting for you! It's getting annoying, Fatty. The tires belong on your car, not your midsection. How can your spirit dwell proudly in an excess of 40 pounds? How can your dance moves come out to play if you can't make it for longer than two hours in those heels?

I'm not mad at you. I'm just impatient. I want you to live your life fully, unapologetically, with your head up and your chin in singular. The warrior you have so long searched for is right there, inside of you. I am her. I am you. Let me take over. I'm stronger than he ever was. And I am stronger than you.

Say "Yes" to bikini summers and a long, radiant life.

Say "No" to pasta and cake. Or, maybe . . . just take one bite.

Love, always, in largeness or a size 2, but come on already!

Skinny Beatrice Badass

Having completed your letter to Not-Thin You, now allow her to write you back. Allow her to tell you what *she* wants to say. Your subconscious mind is delivering the messages you need to hear and the images you need to see. Listen deeply, and write down what you feel is her truth. It's there.

Beatrice continued:

Dear Skinny,

F#@ you.*

It's not easy, sister. It's a daily siege of sliding 180 pounds into jeans that barely button. I know the answers.

I'm having a hard time, okay? I know I'm not really an elephant. Without this unflattering excess million pounds of sadness and fear, all piled unceremoniously on my ass, and thighs, and belly, I am <u>actually</u> a yogi acrobat. A lotus hovering three feet off the ground and spinning somersaults, while gracefully holding up bills-groceries-car payments-<u>life.</u>

But it just so happens that at the moment I am a <u>large</u> yogi, stuck on planet Earth, in flats. Cartwheels are a distant dream. But . . . I hear you. I know he is gone. It's just taking me a minute (30 years long) to fully know that, to fully know that his face is not the face of every man I meet—that I do not need to re-create him, that once was (more than) enough.

This cellulite is my force field, my invisible shield, my insurance policy. Fat Ass = No Possibility of Getting Hurt. Not able to get into a beautiful dress and rock the dance floor means no evil jackass will have the opportunity to get up in this beautiful mess and cause another hurricane, another tornado, a volcanic siege.

Alone in bed with Luda the Greatest Dog Ever to Live + Large Pizza with Extra Sausage and Cheese = Easy and Safe. Beautiful and Sexy means Open for Hurt.

Listen, Skinny Superhero. Give me a minute. I am getting there. I have found the yoga studio, and there are avocados in the fridge. The sun is shining today, and there is work to be done. I am dreaming of one hundred easy sit-ups and that beautiful sheer tank top with the flowers on it.

I'm in, okay?
Jeez, you are a pain in the gigantic ass.
But I love you for always being with(in) me.
In solidarity of spirit, not thigh circumference,
Your Fat Self

Do not underestimate the power of writing these letters. Building this relationship between Thin You and Not-Thin You is the beginning of your reconciliation with a part of yourself that belongs inside, not outside, your castle doors.

Dear God,
Please forgive me
if I have failed to love
every part of Your creation.
Open my eyes that I might see,
soften my heart that I might love,
open my mind that I might understand
every aspect of myself.
Heal my relationship
with all of me,
that I might suffer no more
such violence toward myself.
Please help me, for by myself I cannot win this war.
Please lift me above the battlefield
to the peace that lies beyond.
Thank You, God.
Amen

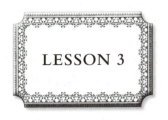

BUILD YOUR ALTAR

In Alcoholics Anonymous, there is the notion of a Higher Power, or God *as you understand Him*. And that is fine for our purposes. It doesn't matter what you call it, as long as you call *on* it. The point is not a name or a word or any religious doctrine or dogma. The point is a spiritual principle that becomes a living reality, affecting both body and soul: that a power greater than the mortal mind, in you but not of you, can do for you what you cannot do for yourself.

Consider what that means to you. You might wish to use your journal pages to write down your thoughts, take a minute to reflect on your spiritual beliefs, or talk to friends or counselors about your ideas. This course is not so much about your relationship to food as it is about your relationship to your Creator. In healing your relationship to Him, you heal your relationship to yourself; and in healing your relationship to yourself, you heal your relationship to everything.

Our goal is that you have a miracle. But a miracle comes from somewhere; it emerges not from your mortal mind but from the mind of God. For the purposes of these 21 lessons, it will be helpful for you to entertain the possibility that

Divine Mind can miraculously heal you. That is all you need do: be willing to consider the possibility that this is true. By opening your mind to the possibility of a miracle, you pave the way for your experience of one.

You have tried many ways to end your food hell, from various food programs to exercise to fasting to who-knows-what. Now I propose that you try something you may or may not have tried before. I suggest that you plant a mustard seed and let God's strength grow within you. "The kingdom of heaven is like a grain of mustard seed that a man took and sowed in his field. It is the smallest of all seeds, but when it has grown it is larger than all the garden plants and becomes a tree" (Matthew 13:31–32).

I suggest you accept this fact: that you cannot beat this problem by yourself. You cannot stop. You have no control over it. It is bigger than you are. If you could have done this by yourself, you would have done so by now.

Your freedom lies in *accepting* that which frightens you most: that you are powerless to stop this problem, to fight it or to fix it . . . your compulsion to eat excessively is stronger than you are . . . you are so tired of this war you have fought against yourself that part of you would rather die than go on.

It's time to surrender the struggle now.

And how does that feel to you? Does it feel like a relief, or does it make you nervous? "What? Surrender? As in, just give up?" you might say. "Are you crazy? How can I give up?! If I give up, I will become truly obese! I might even die! I'll be out of control entirely!"

Yet aren't you out of control now? Exactly what part of you would guide you to *keep up* the fight? This voice that seems to be speaking to you with such concern and wisdom, warning you to keep fighting—is that a power that has proven effective at solving the problem? And if in fact it hasn't, then isn't it time to fire it as your guide?

Your salvation in this area lies not in resisting the truth of your powerlessness before food, but rather in accepting it. For this acceptance leads you straight into the arms of God, however you think of Him or whatever you understand Him to be. You realize, once you accept that your problem is bigger than you are, that perhaps something else is bigger than *it.*

You are now at one of the most important crossroads of your life, as a problem you have dealt with for a long time has reached a climax. Perhaps you feel cornered now, as though you've tried everything and all your efforts are spent. Having depended on your own strength to heal yourself, you have ended up smack-dab back in the center of the wound. You feel checkmated by yourself and beaten by your own ego. All your efforts have been for nothing when confronted by the demonic power of your compulsion to eat excessively.

Yet the very situation that has wounded you can now become that which heals you, if you allow it to take you deep into the mystery of the soul's dependence on the Divine. Do not forget that while your wound is more powerful than your conscious mind, God is more powerful than your wound.

I cannot, but God can! I cannot, but God can! becomes your mantra. And in realizing that the power of your mortal self is small when compared to the power of God, you will no longer need to "puff yourself up" in an effort to make yourself "big enough" to handle your problems. In fact, you will discover the power of true humility, deferring to a power that is greater than your own. God is big enough to handle your problems—*so you need not be.*

It can feel almost personally insulting when you first see that your personal part in making your life run smoothly is so small compared to His. Yet that is exactly the right relationship of mortal to Divine power. In order to end your compulsive eating's reign of terror, you need a power that actually moves through your brain, changes your nervous system, changes your patterns and habits, changes your self-image, changes your thoughts about food, changes your thoughts about your body; and a myriad of other physical, emotional, and psychological factors.

What worldly power could achieve such a total make-over? When you accept the possibility that there might be another way—that perhaps a miracle *could* happen—then you permit your mind to experience one. Something you always intuited but were terrified to admit—that of yourself you don't have what it takes to lose your weight and keep it off permanently—becomes a relief. You don't, but God does.

It is when you allow God to be bigger, that you will allow yourself to become physically smaller. You will begin to give up your burdens when you remember there is someone to give them to.

The weight on your body is nothing compared to the weight on your heart . . . the sadness, the shame, the despair, the weariness. Yet imagine, if only for a moment, that there is a force in the universe that would take your sorrow and shame and all the rest, and simply lift them from your shoulders. You are carrying burdens you were not meant to carry *and do not have to carry.* Your weight is a burden you can now give over. You were created to travel lightly on this planet, with the same sense of relaxed joy that little children have. As soon as you lighten up your mind, your body will lighten up as well.

A small child living in a normal, healthy environment is free and relaxed because he or she assumes that an adult is handling his or her needs. That is meant to be a model for the development of our healthy relationship to the Divine. You are meant to trust the universe like a child trusts an adult. *If,* however, you came to feel as a child that your adult authority figures could *not* be trusted, then you have had a harder time transitioning into a healthy dependence on the ultimate nature of reality. You think you're on your own and have to handle everything by yourself. No wonder you feel heavy. . . .

Consequently, you have had a difficult time processing your emotions. You don't work through them; you hold on to them. You try to stuff them. Problems arise, both conscious and unconscious, and instead of giving them up, you *take them in.* You subconsciously make your body a larger size in order to contain your large problems. You try to create a big enough container to carry all your issues, when you shouldn't be carrying all those issues to begin with!

Perhaps you are someone who feels a need to sabotage yourself when things get too good. Perhaps you've made a subconscious decision that you should allow yourself only *this* much success, or *this* much money, or *this* much physical beauty or happiness. And why? It could be a lot of reasons: perhaps you grew up afraid to break through barriers that your parents didn't break through, or were ashamed of being successful when those around you weren't, or were concerned that you'd lose someone's love or approval if you dared to have the life you really wanted.

It doesn't matter why your own invisible barrier exists, that point past which the subconscious alarm starts blaring, "Uh-oh! Too much good! Too much good! You mustn't go there! Go back!" As in, *go back into that limited condition where you belong. Don't you dare break free. If you break through that barrier, all hell will break loose!* But in front of that barrier is where hell in fact has already broken loose. . . .

An overwhelming urge to overeat reflects the hidden barrier you erected within your mind; you are invited to cross that barrier now and to make a run for freedom. Imagine God Himself, in whatever form He appears to you, walking up to the barrier and smashing it. It is the barrier itself that is the root of your problem. It is not enough to control your appetite; true healing involves dissolving the barrier, removing the false thinking that has kept you bound.

Let's now ask God to free you of the mental limitations that exist within you like petty tyrants. There is no way to surrender your weight without surrendering your subconscious belief that you're better off weighing too much. If you're subconsciously convinced that being heavy is a *safer* zone than being thin, then of course your primal urge to protect yourself will make sure you stay heavy. You'll feel a subconscious need to sabotage your greater good.

Sometimes we're tempted to cap our good, afraid that what happens when the cap is removed is too chaotic, too out-of-control a process. But the life we live at the behest of our control mechanisms—whether expressed as an obsessive urge to eat or an obsessive refusal to eat—is the life that is out of control. Trying to keep down your feelings, your gorgeousness, your success, your *life force,* you are seeking to put a cap on life itself. And this cannot be done. No matter how much you try to abort the process, life happens. It will unfold beautifully, or it will unfold less than beautifully. But it will unfold.

And this is a good thing. For all that life energy coming at you is not a threat, but a gift; it's not a curse, but a blessing. Your alternative to trying to cap what cannot be capped anyway is to *allow* it, to stand before the wellspring of life not seeking to tamp it down, but rather enjoying its delights. The deeper delights you are seeking are not found in food, but rather in living fully. Don't resist the flow of life;

relax into the middle of it, and marvel at the ever-unfolding miracle which is life itself. God knows how to be God, and will show you—if you allow Him to—the awesomeness of creation as it manifests in and through you.

Spiritually, your wanting to lose weight is not a desire to become less of yourself, but rather a desire to become *more* of your *true* self. And you remember who you truly are when you remember Who created you. By reestablishing your right relationship to your Source, you reestablish your right relationship to yourself—in mind *and* in body. You are a being both created by love and at home in love. Your deepest desire is not for food, but for the experience of home. Your deepest desire is not for food, but for love.

Love is both the creator of the universe and the order of the universe. We vastly underestimate the seismic rupture caused by the slightest deviation from love. Every moment of unconscious eating is a moment when you are starving from a lack of healthy self-love, and struggling to find it elsewhere. Just as a child in the womb receives its nourishment directly from its mother, so we are to receive our true nourishment directly from the Divine. In reestablishing your relationship with your Divine Source, you will once again receive Divine nourishment. As your connection to love is repaired, you'll be freed from your compulsion to seek love from a source that only dishes out self-hate.

You were taught to be self-reliant, and of course that is a good thing. But your dependence on God is not the abdication of responsibility; it is the ultimate taking of responsibility. It doesn't make you less powerful to acknowledge a Higher Power; it makes you *more* powerful, because it gives you access to the power of faith.

Faith is an aspect of consciousness; there is no such thing as a faithless person. Right now, you have plenty of faith . . . faith that you'll eat too much, no matter what you do. Faith that you'll never lose the weight and really keep it off. Faith that overeating is your only true friend, even though you know it's anything but your friend. The real question is, do you have more faith in the power of your problem or in the power of a miracle to solve it?

Let's try tweaking your faith a bit here. Believe, even if only for just a moment, that God will work a miracle in your life. Try having faith in *that*. He will take away your inappropriate and excessive desires for food; He will remove your false appetites and return your body to its natural wisdom; He will restore your life to purpose and joy. And if you can't do that—if you can't summon up the faith—then, if only for a moment, lean on mine.

The problem is not that we're not believers; most of us are. The problem is that we too often keep our "belief" or even our "faith" separate from the rest of our lives. As though spirituality is some separate corner of life, distinct from our bodies or relationships or work lives or any other practical concerns.

"God has enough to think about," people often say, as though we shouldn't bother Him with our petty problems. But there is no spot in the universe that isn't filled, infused, permeated, and lifted up by the Divine. Your Creator can't *be* left out, except in your thinking. And wherever He is left out in your thinking, He can't help you. Let Him help you lose weight, and He will.

At about this point, your fear-mind might be starting to disparage these lessons. In your overeating, fear has found in you a perversely comfortable home, and it will not move out of its lair so easily. With every step forward, it will try to lure you back. "This is nonsense." "This can't work." "God has nothing to do with your weight." Such are the kinds of ammunition it will use to make sure that no matter what else you do, you will not give this course a chance.

For something in your thinking has begun to expand, and the spirit of fear *will have none of that.* "Whoa, slow down!" fear will say. Or "This is a waste of time." Or the pseudointellectual one: "Faith isn't *rational!*" Well, neither is a loving embrace, but no one would doubt its power.

Fear is a psychic tyrant that has no intention of letting its slave go free. It will say whatever it needs to say to confuse your thinking and pervert your appetites. It will always seek to preserve itself, and it doesn't mind your being spiritual or religious as long as you don't actually *apply it to your life* too much. It doesn't mind your going to church, as long as you are *fat* and going to church. You are to do what it says, how and when it says to do it. And nothing—not your best intentions, your willpower, or your self-discipline—has the power to overrule its authority. Only God does.

Let us increase your faith in *that.*

The work of this lesson is to build an altar to the Divine. You will build a spiritual altar in your heart, and a physical altar in your home.

Fear already has an altar—it's called your kitchen. It has cabinets and a refrigerator, drawers of packaged goods, and forks and knives and spoons. It has all those things, plus counters, a sink, and more. It is the headquarters for many of your fears.

Let us now establish another headquarters: a headquarters for love.

With this lesson, your assignment is to create a place in your home that will remind you that love, *not fear,* is the true power in your life. Every time you visit your altar, it will fortify love's power in your mind. And the more love fills your mind, the more miracles will fill your life.

Look around you and consider what area of your home might best be used for your altar. Your altar should both celebrate and support the power of Divine love. Seated next to it should be a chair for reading inspirational material, praying, and meditating. The altar should include a surface on which to place beautiful or meaningful objects that remind you of Spirit. This book, of course . . . and pictures, holy books, statues, fresh flowers, prayer beads, sacred objects . . . all are examples of appropriate items to be placed upon your altar. As you go through this course—indeed, as you move through the journey of your entire life—it would be good to make your altar a continuous expression of your devotion to God. This dedicated space reminds you to bow down to love and love only. And every time you write in your journal, you should return it to your altar.

"Love the Lord thy God with all thy heart, with all thy soul, with all thy might" is the First Commandment . . . and why? Because it is the key to right living. We should focus on Divine will because if we don't, then our focus will be given over to something else. That something else is neurosis, pathology, compulsion, and fear. In our separation from the thoughts of love, blind to the true Source of our good, we look for love in all the wrong places. *That* is idolatry. Eating has become a false idol for you.

On any given day when you feel triggered, when you are deeply drawn to the ritualistic dance of self-hatred that is overeating, you will have more power to resist if on that day you have already experienced the power of your altar . . . if you have already prayed and given thanks to God. For having already bowed before the power of the Divine, you will be far less tempted to bow before the power of your compulsion to overeat.

Having begun to build your altar to love, let's begin to tear down your altar to fear. First, walk into your kitchen and pray that it be home to love and love only.

Dear God,
I dedicate this room to You.
May only love prevail here.
May fear have power no more,
in my heart, in my body, or in my house.
Amen

Also, there is a Native American tradition called "smudging" that you might find useful. It involves gathering some sage and burning it over a bowl—in this case, in your kitchen. Along with prayer, this herbal ritual will help clear out your dysfunctional appetites. The two will purify the room of compulsive energies still hanging in the air, the psychic leftovers of one who used to bow like a slave before the altar to fear. *That person is no longer who you are.* Even though the ghost of your former self might appear to taunt you, do not let this scare you. You have remembered what is holy, and what is not holy can no longer hurt you.

I suggest you rid your kitchen of all trigger foods, for they can still harm you as long as you do not have the will to resist their temptation. If the thought occurs to you that you are throwing away good food that costs real money, remind yourself that too much unhealthy food could in fact cost you your life. Fill your kitchen instead with colorful, nutritious foods; enlist family and friends to help you in this process, if you need their support. Get rid of all that is unhealthy, and make your kitchen a sacred place.

Moving back to your new altar—your altar to the power of love—allow yourself, while sitting before it, to imbibe the energies of Spirit. Books, music, letter writing, pictures . . . anything that helps build the thought-forms and feelings of a more beautiful life. Even books about food are fine, as long as they are about wise and healthy eating.

You might take the opportunity to expand your reading to a powerful set of principles: the Twelve Steps of Overeaters Anonymous (OA). Whether you are an addict or a compulsive eater—who, while not addicted to a specific food, is still unable to control your desire to eat excessively—the principles of OA carry a universal wisdom that has saved the lives of millions.

The steps are universal adages that speak to anyone dealing with an addiction, and the first three encapsulate the meaning of spiritual surrender: that as an addict you must admit that you are powerless before your problem, that only God is powerful enough to restore you to sanity, and that as an addict you must turn your will and life over to the care of God as you understand Him.

Addiction represents the place where one's sanity is overruled. No matter what you do—no matter how much you diet or exercise—as long as there is that place in your brain where your sanity flips over like a breaker switch, then even your best efforts will seem for naught. This then makes your life unmanageable. It is as though there is a place where you are always rendered powerless, no matter how powerful you might be in other ways.

Only you can say if you are an addict. Addiction is more than compulsion: it demands abstinence from particular items (at least temporarily), whether they be made of sugar, white flour, or refined carbohydrates; or specific binge foods. Coming to terms with the idea that you are an addict is a huge thing, and should be treated with proper respect. Respect for your grief over the pain you have already caused yourself. Respect for the disappointment you feel at knowing you must abstain from certain substances in order to be free. Respect for the pain you are in now, as you allow yourself to open to many thoughts and feelings only now beginning to surface.

This is not a journey you should take alone. Perhaps you have a group of like-minded friends who in suffering what you have suffered can share the pain and power of this journey with you. A solitary path will only give more power to fear, while walking this path with others will give it the power and blessing of love. If you feel drawn to this course and want to dive into it more deeply, perhaps you have friends who wish to practice the lessons with you. Connecting deeply to other people *is* a connection to the Divine.

Only the Divine is more powerful than fear, rendering powerless that which has rendered *you* powerless. Only Divine Mind can restore you to your right mind. Every thought that you yourself can manage your addiction, or get on top of it or make it go away, is a thought that will only lead you in time straight back into your addictive behavior.

That is why the message here is not "Don't think so much about food." The message is "Think more about God." Through a powerful shift in your relationship to God, your relationship with food will begin to shift as well. But turning your life over to the Divine is more than a kinda-sorta-sometimes thing. It is a full-throttle willingness to let go of everything—every thought, every pattern, and every desire—that blocks love from entering you and extending through you. It is not enough to just transform some of your thoughts, or even your body. You'll get free, and remain free, only if you are willing to transform your life.

You will now begin to see how problematic situations that have little or nothing to do with food have *everything* to do with food, if they represent your blocks to love. It's a subtle but very powerful shift from "I turn this situation or that into the hands of God," to, as they say in AA, "I turn *my life and will* over to the care of God." Unless your entire life is turned over, and not just your excessive eating, then your compulsion will always find fertile soil in which to grow back.

Fear is like a thief with endless patience, casually circling your house in the belief that you will ultimately be careless enough to leave one of the doors unlocked. It will simply hide and wait. "It's okay. So what if you've been eating and exercising so well for the last month. I'll just wait till you get stressed over that situation at work, and I'll put some sugar in front of you while you're going through it." It is that sly, that insidious, and that vicious. Your job is to post enough angels around your house that the thief cannot get in.

Reflection and Prayer

Closing your eyes, see your body infused with light. Every cell is filled with a golden elixir poured forth from Divine Mind. Angels are gathered around you as you allow yourself to release yourself fully into the field of the Divine.

Hold this image for at least five minutes. Breathe out your burdens, and breathe in love's miraculous power. See light pouring into your body. Continue to do this visualization, using it when any problem occurs to you.

The point is to not just release your *weight* to God, but to surrender *everything* to Him. And *everything* includes your body. For a minimum of five minutes, allow Divine Mind to have full and total access to your physical self. The imagery that emerges from this experience is the beginning of a process by which fear's hold on your body imagery will be fundamentally, and ultimately permanently, dismantled.

When you walk to the kitchen, see Him walking with you. When you take a bite, surrender it to Him. Even if you overeat, surrender the experience to Spirit as you do so. "Dear God, I surrender this experience to you. Amen." Do not fight yourself. Simply cleave to God.

God is not your judge but your healer. It's not as though He's been unaware of your patterns, or of your suffering. He has simply been waiting for this day, when you would invite Him to enter and to do what only He can do.

Dear God,
My eyes have been opened to the nature of my disease.
I am powerless before food, and I realize that now.
I surrender to You both my pain and my compulsion.
Please do for me what I cannot do for myself.
Dear God, please overpower my false appetites
and cast out my fear.
I thank You for Your love,
which I know has blessed me.
I thank You for Your blessing,
which I know will heal me.
And may my healing, dear God,
be of use to others
in whatever way that You direct.
Amen

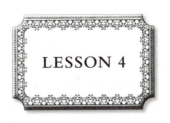

INVOKE THE REAL YOU

You have a physical set of eyes and a spiritual set of eyes. With your physical eyes you see the material world, but there is more to life than the material world.

With your spiritual eyes, you see beyond appearances. You see into the realm of Divine possibility, and by *seeing* a new possibility, you invoke it. Instead of allowing appearances to determine what you think is real, you can decide what you think is real; by doing so, you can cause a change in what you see.

Once you see who you really are, you will permit the real you to come forth.

This is neither theory nor theology. It's neither symbol nor metaphor nor hopeful fantasy. This lesson will be as real in your experience as you choose it to be, and to the extent that it is real for you, its effects will be real in your life.

The real you is neither fat nor skinny. The real you is not a body at all, but rather a spirit . . . an energy . . . an idea in the Mind of God. The real you is a being of light, and therefore has no material density. As you align more and more with this truth of your being, this higher reality will permeate all aspects of your life. *The more you identify with the light of your being, the lighter you will feel.* You will materialize a lighter body when you have a more light-filled mind.

Fear literally weighs you down, but love en-lightens you. Any subject, energy, circumstance, thought, feeling, interpretation, perspective, goal, substance, or relationship that fosters fear in you is something that feeds your compulsion, because compulsion is your fallback position in the presence of fear. The question is: What are you afraid of?

The first answer that suggests itself is that you are afraid of being even heavier, of never getting your eating under control, of never getting this monkey off your back and so forth. But beneath that fear is an even deeper one. Your deepest fear isn't of being fat; your deepest fear is of being thin. *Your deepest fear is of being beautiful.*

For many people, compulsive eating is tied to a fear of sex and of being sexy. In particular, the number of women whose excess weight can be almost directly traced to sexual abuse is significant. *When I was beautiful, I was molested.* Or, *When I was beautiful, I was raped.* Or, *When I'm beautiful, I don't know how to handle the sexual attention.* Such thoughts run rampant through the minds of many who are overweight, men as well as women.

If the idea of being skinny frightens you, there's no point trying to get rid of what your subconscious mind has created as your security blanket. For subconsciously, you will not let it go. There are many ways to hide, and weight is one of them. Some people hide behind a wall of weight as a refuge from the risk of inappropriate or even criminal sexual contact.

If these dark shadows of sexuality lurk behind your fear of being thin, then the way to disperse those shadows is not to deny your sexuality, but to purify it of error. Sometimes that means forgiving someone else, and sometimes it means forgiving yourself.

Certainly feminism has helped empower women, the women's movement has liberated us to actualize more of our human potential, and the modern view of women has helped us right injustices like the subjugation and oppression of females. At the same time, however, there are certain cultural attitudes more endemic to former times that served us well, the absence of which has left us exposed to energies no woman should be exposed to. *Freedom* and *license* are two very different words, and the sexual freedom of the 1960s— while in many ways a wonderful form of liberation indeed— carried with it, as most things do, some hidden potential for misuse.

Modesty is not just some old-fashioned we-don't-need-this-anymore value; it is a spiritual energy that dignifies and protects female sexuality from both abuse by men and misuse by women. Casual sex is not just wrong for some moralistic reason; it's wrong because it violates something profound and extraordinary by cheapening its value. "Starting too young" is not just wrong because of societal attitudes; it's wrong because the brain of a young teenager (and certainly those younger than that) is not developed enough, and the personality of that young of a person is not experienced enough, to integrate such a powerful experience in the most meaningful way. We have been left exposed over the last few decades to a hell-posing-as-heaven of sexual license, leaving us feeling not so much liberated as unprotected. Many walls were torn down that we then made subconscious and dysfunctional efforts to build back up. Packing on pounds is one of them.

As your fear is reduced, your body will reduce itself. When you no longer fear the world so much, you will be more comfortable dwelling in it. Dwelling more comfortably in the world, you will begin to dwell more comfortably in your own skin. And dwelling more comfortably in your own skin, you will subconsciously create a more comfortable body.

If you feel afraid of the world, you feel a perverse comfort in a body that keeps the world at a distance. And that is where the real you comes in. The real you loves the world and doesn't *want* to keep it at a distance. You are here to love the world and for the world to love you. The real you doesn't perceive that fact within a sexual context, but within a spiritual one. The purity of your spirituality heals the toxicity of any sexual impurity in your past.

Your real self is eternally innocent and eternally chaste. Nothing you have ever done and *nothing that anyone has ever done to you* could make imperfect what God created perfect. What God has created is both changeless and forever. The goodness and purity of your essential self is guaranteed for all time. And the more you make conscious contact with that purity, the more quickly dysfunctional thoughts, toxic shame, and other buried feelings that might have arisen from sexual violation will begin to dissolve and disappear forever.

In Divine Mind, you exist as a Divine image. And that is the truth of who you are. That image has a twin within the physical world, and she is waiting to be born. Her existence expresses itself as you at your healthiest, happiest, and most creative. Your body at its perfect shape and weight *already exists* within Divine Mind, the realm of pure possibility, because all that is perfect dwells in Divine possibility. Your perfect weight, as an expression of the real you, is not just a vague hope dangling out in the universe somewhere— rather, it is a Divine imprint gestating within you. As an overweight person, you have given birth to the body of your suffering; it's time now to give birth to the body of your joy.

There is no wall around the real you, but that doesn't mean she is unprotected. She is protected by a mantle of blessing. Her weight is down, but her sexual energy reads "Don't even think about it" to anyone but appropriate partners. Having forgiven herself and anyone who transgressed against her, she has learned her lesson and healed her heart. There is no need or subconscious urge to attract a similar situation again. Having been herself reminded of her fundamental virtue, others are automatically reminded of it as well when in her presence. Only those who are worthy will come courting, and only those who are worthy will be invited into her court.

The real you is not afraid of being thin, because she knows the real world is not a dangerous place and the real world is where she lives. The real world is not material but spiritual. The real world is not chaotic or licentious or violent or fearful; the real world is simply love.

Your beauty—and every one of us is beautiful when we allow ourselves to be—is a gift from God. It is a blessing bestowed upon you and meant to emanate from you. It is not a source of shame or falsehood or illusion; it is a source of joy and blessing. The world is not made better by your hiding out, spiritually or physically. The same God who created roses created you. The real you, like the rose itself, is naturally and unself-consciously beautiful. And the world is more beautiful because of it.

A spiritual practice is your bridge back to the real you and to the real world. Through prayer, meditation, forgiveness, and compassion, you make conscious contact with your spiritual self, your most beautiful self, and hasten the process of your healing.

As you allow Divine Mind access to your thinking, you allow it access to your body as well. Spirit *moves* things, including biological forces. And it *removes* things as well. With this lesson, you ask Divine Mind to remove any fear you have of being who you really are. Learning to be comfortable with your own magnificence—your own reality as a child of God—is the goal of any spiritual quest, including this one.

The real you is like a file in a computer that's not currently downloaded. It exists; it just hasn't been brought up on your screen yet. And that's because it hasn't been chosen. Fear rather than love has been doing your choosing, but as you do the lessons in this course, you will begin to choose differently. The more you align with the real you, the real you will make more of your choices. And the real you will always choose love.

The choice to eat wisely is not important simply because it leads to an arguably more attractive you; it isn't important simply because it offers the possibility of a smaller dress size; it isn't even important simply because it's healthier. It's important because it's an act of love. It's a way that you feed who you want to be—the healthier you, the more beautiful you, the more comfortable you, the happier you. And what you feed, you will call forth. You are not truly feeding yourself when you eat excessively; in fact, you are withholding sustenance from yourself when you overeat, for in so doing, you are withholding love.

One of the ways you love yourself is by permitting yourself to want what you want. One of the reasons people consume *anything* too much is because they don't consume other things *enough*. You tend to take in too much material substance when you are starving yourself of spiritual substance.

Overeating is an act of spiritual starvation, and one of the things the overeater often starves herself of is the natural right to dream. Invoking the real you begins with expanding your imagination, allowing yourself to want what you really want. You have as much of a right to your dreams as does any other person. And if you won't let a thinner you live in your imagination, then there's no way you'll let her live in your body.

Perhaps you have a picture of yourself when your weight was what you want now, or you can get a picture from a book or magazine that represents your desired look. Make sure, however, that if you do use an image of another person, that you put a picture of *your own face* on it—otherwise, this exercise can be used to depress you rather than heal you. These lessons are not about your wanting to be someone else; they're about your learning to manifest your own best self. And your best self has an appreciation for the beauty of this world, including your own. Beauty and sensuality are gifts of nature, and if anyone or anything has sullied them in your mind, then it is time to heal that now.

The sensual aspect of your body is a spiritual gift; experiencing it is part of the glory of being human. Deep down, you want the experience of a waistline; you want the experience of a lighter body. You want the experience of self-love in its totality.

It's not just your right but also your purpose on Earth to become the person you long to be. You don't long to be a victim; you long to be good, healthy, and creative. You long to feel the fun of a fit body and the joy of being able to run around with your children and grandchildren. You long to have a non-obsessive relationship with food, and you long to look in the mirror and like what you see.

No one but you is denying yourself these experiences, and your facing that fact—that *you* are cruel to *you*, that *you* are withholding from *you*, that *you* are harming *you*—is both horrifying and liberating to look squarely in the eye. Have you bludgeoned yourself enough yet, do you think? Have you figured out yet what you did to deserve this? And are you ready for a miracle?

Regardless of your weight, you might not have the build of a supermodel. And that's okay. When your body is toned and at a weight that is healthy and right for you, it's beautiful. If you put a picture of a supermodel on your refrigerator—with your face instead of hers—then that's fine. You're not self-destructively setting your sights on an unrealistic goal; you're simply allowing your heart to own what it really wants.

Your desire is a good thing, not an enemy. You're not diminishing your seriousness by celebrating your physicality. You're not giving in to some chauvinist fantasy by saying, "Yes, damn it, I want that!" You're not trying to escape your life; you're trying at last to claim your life!

The more you embrace the image of a beautiful body and emotionally permit yourself to desire one, the more your subconscious mind will make one manifest. "I shouldn't want that," "I can never have that," or "I don't want that anyway" is *not* the instruction your subconscious mind should be receiving when you look at Beyoncé.

Perhaps you carry ugly pictures in your head—pictures of a fat stomach, huge thighs, a double chin, and so forth. These might be exaggerated and distorted images and not how others even see you, but they have led to negative self-talk that both attacks these images and reinforces them at the same time. Now, by putting your face atop a picture of a beautiful body—whether or not it's even representative of your body type—you have the chance to project the real you into the world, usurping an old, ugly self-image and flooding your mind with a new, gorgeous one.

You are not comparing and contrasting your body with that of a thin person, leading only to the seesaw of alternating motivation and despair. You are not trying to be someone else; you are simply invoking the archetype of the beautiful human form. You are embracing the beauty that is absolutely your Divine right, every bit as much as it belongs to anyone else. Someone with a beautiful body is not revealing what is his or hers alone; he or she is revealing an archetypal energy. You are invoking energy as an absolute, an aspect of the Divine within us all.

Take any action that will further this process. Make copies of that picture of your face atop a beautiful body and put them in various places around your home. Make sure you put them on your refrigerator, a cabinet in your kitchen, and your bathroom mirror. Make your kitchen and bedroom a visual homage to these images. And do not forget to place the picture on your altar. No matter what you think of these pictures on a conscious level, or what those around you may think of them, they are imprinting themselves on your subconscious mind.

Every time you look at that picture, you're inviting your inner thin person to come forth. Your "inner thin" doesn't represent a false value, a superficial or shallow image created by fashion magazines just to taunt you. Your desire to be thin is a valid desire . . . the desire to be healthy, to be light on your feet, to be comfortable in your skin, to have fun with clothes, to enjoy your body, to be sensual, and to be free of compulsion.

You have within you an internal guidance system. It is perfectly calibrated to keep the systems of your body in working order. It guides your breathing, brain functioning, digestion, and so forth. And when you were an infant, it guided your hunger and desire for food. Your guidance system in this area has admittedly been knocked out of working order, but there is nothing inherently permanent about this disorder. When your *spiritual guidance system* is back in order, your physical guidance system will fall back into place as well. This might not happen immediately, but it will happen. Manifesting your perfect weight is simply a natural result of realigning with your true self.

Remember: your beauty already exists in the mind of God, and the more you claim it as already existing, the more quickly it will materialize. You have explored the zone of a heavier existence; now explore the zone of a lighter one. Think of yourself as the most gorgeous god or goddess, thin and radiant. Get to know this aspect of yourself. Relate to your true self where your true self resides: in the inner temple of your heart. And inevitably your true self will come forth. Your body today is a product of yesterday's thinking; as your thoughts change today, your body will be different tomorrow.

Don't wait till she materializes before you relate to your truest self. Relate to her now. Inhabit her now.

Write to her now.

Go to your journal pages and write a letter to Thin You, just as in Lesson 2 you wrote to Not-Thin You. Tell her what you think of her, and if necessary, why you've been scared of her.

Then allow her to write back to you. Allow her to tell you what *she* needs, in order to come forth.

An example might be:

Dear Thin Me,

Well, I haven't seen you in so long that I don't even know for sure if you exist. I mean, I guess you exist as a possibility—if that's really an existence. But you're not the body I see when I wake up each day, I know that for sure. And I think my life might be better if I didn't even hope to ever see you. I don't know whether I should hate you or love you, but I know in my heart that I wish I was you. I really do.

For whatever it's worth, I'm sorry that I make it so hard for you.

I understand that I've made it hard for you to appear, and that I have done more to hurt you than you have done to hurt me. I wish I knew how to be thin and stay thin, but I have had a serious problem with my weight, as you know, and I haven't been able to do any better than I have done.

I am hoping that God will help me so I can allow you to come forth and be the body I want. I give up any thoughts or feelings that make it harder for you to happen, and I am praying for a miracle.

Love,
Me

And would she not write back something along this line:

Dear Not-Thin Me,
Whenever you are ready, I'll be there.
See you soon.
Love,
Me

Return your journal to the altar when you are done. This will add devotional energy to the work you are doing.

Reflection and Prayer

With your eyes closed, see within the middle of your mind a little ball of golden light. Now see within this light yourself as you are now. See your body as it is now, your weight as it is now, your entire being as it is now.

Now see a ball of light form within the center of your chest. Watch the light expand into a golden glow that covers your entire body, ultimately casting out the vision of your physical self.

Now see within this light a new body begin to form: the body of your true self, an image both radiant and Divine.

Ask Divine Mind to place within you a visualization of your perfect self . . . giving . . . forgiving . . . caring . . . assured . . . whole . . . fearless . . . and filled with love. What does that body look like? It might be someone who is very thin; it might be someone who is not thin, but rather full-bodied yet healthy and toned. When you have acquired that kind of internal fullness, whatever it may be, your external self cannot help but be beautiful.

When Divine Mind places this image within you, it will fill your soul. It will be like some astral, energetic body that already exists. It has not yet been downloaded into physical manifestation, but it exists in the spiritual ethers. It exists in the realm of infinite possibility. It exists in the realm of pure potential. And you are shifting your sense of reality from a narrow-minded focus on what exists in the physical world to the broad-minded embrace of what exists in the realm of Spirit, for what exists in the realm of Spirit is in fact *more real*.

Perhaps the fear-mind will taunt you. "This is three-dimensional reality, Buster. This is *real*. You may as well *accept* it." But for the purposes of this visualization, know that *you don't have to accept it*. The masters of metaphysical transformation have realized this secret of the ages: that the physical dimension is just one dimension, and it is the follower, not the leader, of the others. Mind, spirit, and imagination rule—if you will allow them to.

Own the power of your imagination. Do not be limited *in any way at all* by what you think of as possible, probable, or logical.

You want a beautiful body? Go for it. Imagine it. Allow the image to permeate your consciousness. Embrace it. Do not hold it at bay. You want a bodybuilder's physique? Go for it. Embrace it. Own it. Open up the prison of your mind, and for once, with full permission given by yourself to yourself, *allow yourself to want what you really want*. If you ask yourself what you want and the answer is a second bowl of ice cream or a second slice of cake, then ask yourself what you *really* want. You will find that as you own your desire for the body of your dreams, your desire for that second bowl of ice cream will begin to wane.

Allow yourself to be—with all your real desires and hopes and dreams—and see the perfect shape of things to come. Breathe in the images and feel the joy of their presence. Allow God in all His mysterious power to do the rest.

Dear God,
Please deliver me to
my own true self.
Please make of my body
a perfect container
for who You created me to be.
And teach me how to live within it
in happiness and peace.
Amen

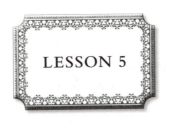

START A LOVE AFFAIR WITH FOOD

You probably read this chapter title over a couple of times thinking that you'd caught a typo. Perhaps you thought I must have meant *end* your love affair with food, not start one. But nope, you read it right the first time. It's time for you to *start* a real love affair with food.

What you've had up to this point has been an obsessive relationship, and an obsessive relationship is not love. Whether with a substance or with a person, an obsessive relationship is a dance of the wounded . . . a carnival of pain . . . but not a real love affair, *because there is no love there.* To think you need food that you don't really need, to practically inhale food, to crave food, to obsess about food, to binge on and then alternately avoid food, to control food and need to be rigid around it—none of these bespeak a love affair. Pain and compulsion and self-hate are not love.

The true lover of food is able to take time with it. She can *savor* food, and non-neurotically delight in it. She can chew it thoroughly and actually taste it. She can eat without guilt and stop eating without too great an effort. She can celebrate how food is contributing to her health. She can wonder at it and appreciate its beauty. She can linger over a fruit stand and study the curves of a pear. She can gaze at a pomegranate and feel awe at the fact that thousands of years ago, people ate these, too. She can shop for groceries without wondering if anyone is watching her or judging her. She can gaze at a pretty bunch of grapes and consider whether she'd prefer them in her stomach or in a crystal bowl on her table. She can take one bite of something delicious, ecstatically breathe in the taste, *and* enjoy waiting before taking another bite. For her, the spaces in between each bite are part of the joy of her experience.

No, the compulsive overeater is no lover of food. When it comes to your enjoyment of eating, your best days are not behind you but ahead of you.

The eating patterns of an overeater are chaotic, fearful, furtive, and out of control. And yet, these dysfunctional patterns are not your deeper problem. They are *symptoms* of the problem. Your deeper problem is the hysteria in your gut—the silent, traumatized shriek of "I'm empty! Fill me! I'm empty! Fill me!"—the irrational and irresistible energy that has wormed its way into your brain, stationed itself in your nervous system, and won't let go until you've eaten the whole thing. This course is a plan in dissolving your hysteria and filling your emptiness by replacing it with love.

Years ago, after a spate of horrifying incidents in which high-school students perpetrated acts of violence against teachers and classmates, I noticed an interesting but, I thought, disturbing kind of discipline imposed at my daughter's school. All of a sudden the students had not five minutes between class but only two. Passing notes in class was punishable by serious time in detention. Outdoor activities of all kinds were forbidden, and "downtime" of any sort was also verboten.

I lobbied the school administration, arguing that while I myself worked hard all day, every once in a while I needed to get up from my desk, stretch, do something silly for five minutes, go get some air . . . take a *break!* Kids are human and need that, too!

In encountering the school's resistance to my argument, I realized what had gone on here. This school—and perhaps others as well—had come up with a plan to prevent and discourage negative socialization by suppressing any socialization whatsoever. Don't let kids meet each other; something awful might happen! Don't let them form relationships; they might hurt each other! Don't let them relax; they might use the time to hatch some awful plan! *So, what is the plan here?* I thought. *Train them to be dehumanized zombies and then all will be well?*

My daughter left that school soon thereafter, but what stayed in my mind was the odd irrationality of trying to keep kids separate from each other at school. The answer to antisocial behavior among our children is not that we suppress socialization, but that we teach and model *positive* socialization for them. For me, that's a really big "Duuuhh!"

So it is with dysfunctional eating. The solution to overeating is obviously not to deny yourself food altogether; the answer is not to deny yourself at all. You don't need to forget food, run away from food, deny yourself food, or avoid food. And the last thing you need to do if you want to stop thinking obsessively about food is to tell yourself not to think about it! Doing so is an invitation for such thoughts to overwhelm you.

Food is not only your problem, it is also your teacher. It is a reflection of an even deeper problem, an opportunity and an invitation to face that which underlies your compulsive eating. Your only real problem—everyone's only real problem—is a separation from Divine Mind. Every step taken with love in mind is a step back to who you really are.

This course aims to put genuine love back into your relationship with food: not counterfeit love, not substitute love, but genuine love. Love and gratitude that food nourishes and sustains you. Love and gratitude that meals can build bonds among families and friends. Love and gratitude that food is something you have the right to enjoy, once you learn to relate to it with Divine detachment.

Detachment means that you can take it or leave it; you can enjoy food if you're hungry, but you can leave it alone if you're not. Love, as always, is the key to making things right. By learning to love food, you will stop obsessing about it. And the obsession, not the food, is your actual problem.

Obsession, whether toward a substance or a person, occurs when you're open to giving and yet don't know how to receive. You keep grasping for more because you're not feeling anything coming back. As a child, perhaps, nothing *was* coming back, so now you keep trying to get more of something you're already convinced isn't really there. As you build a relationship with food that *does* give back, you'll begin to experience a relationship in which love has replaced obsession.

The only way to attain healthy neutrality toward food is by learning to love it, and the only food you can really love is food that loves you back.

Does a hot-fudge sundae love you, do you think? It's true that it can give you a momentary high, but so can crystal meth. For me, a special charge from hot-fudge sundaes was connected to the fact that when I was a child, my mother would always take me to Howard Johnson's for a sundae to celebrate things like making a good grade or winning a contest at school. Unfortunately, my brain was then imprinted with the message that big wins should be accompanied by a hot-fudge sundae. It took me years to disconnect from that, and only recently did it occur to me that my mother came up with this celebratory ritual as an excuse to indulge *her* desire for ice cream! (Once you're a mother yourself, you understand your own mother so much better. . . .)

No, hot-fudge sundaes do not love me and they do not love you. They are full of sugar and processed chemicals that bring us anything but love. Those things feed cancer, increase cholesterol, decrease growth hormones, weaken eyesight, interfere with protein absorption, cause food allergies, contribute to diabetes and cardiovascular disease, impair the structure of DNA, create difficulty concentrating, reduce defenses against infectious diseases, lead to osteoporosis, and more. I wouldn't call any of those things *love*.

At the same time, this is not to say that eating a hot-fudge sundae is forbidden for the rest of your life. It's simply to say that as you evolve to your highest sense of self, you won't even *want* to eat a whole hot-fudge sundae; the experience will no longer feel like love to you.

Foods that love you are those that contribute to your well-being. From fruits to vegetables to whole grains, they make your body strong, fight illness, produce great skin, and keep you functioning normally. Vegetables make brain cells grow and function correctly, fruits provide healthy sugar and give you energy, and whole grains can help reduce the risk of cancer and cardiovascular disease. And in today's world, there are more and more ways to find healthy food that is truly tasty. There might be healthier stores and restaurants you pass by frequently that you just never thought of going into . . . and now is the time.

Your problem may not be that you eat so often, but that you do not eat well. Particularly in today's world, while it's easy to eat poorly, it's unnecessary. Today we're in the midst of a food revolution, and that is very good news for the compulsive overeater.

Restaurants now feature the best in nutritious, organic, even vegan, meals. And even when they don't, you can learn to order from a menu in a way that benefits you. Beautiful magazines feature healthy recipes and food displays. Raw food, organic produce, and other optimal food choices abound. Is it always easy, convenient, or inexpensive to make wise food choices? Perhaps not. But let's be very clear: it isn't easy, convenient, or inexpensive to be a food addict either.

Once you know what it is and how to do it, healthy eating is not a punishment but a reward. It's not time for you to give something up so much as it is time for you to take something on. It isn't time to deny yourself but rather a time to gift yourself.

It's sad to realize, but people who spend the most time with food tend to *not* be those taking cooking classes, learning creative recipes, or even eating the best meals. Even if the overeater is going to a fine restaurant in the evening, the chances are good she will have stuffed herself with so much junk food by late afternoon that the actual succulence of eating a good dinner and truly enjoying it will be denied her. By the time she eats the meal, she'll be feeding her psychological appetite, perhaps, but not her stomach, because it's already full. When it comes to the actual joy of eating, the overeater tends to be *deprived*.

It's time to change that. Let's begin your love affair with food.

This lesson comes with assignments, and all that matters is that you do them. Even if you're still eating unwisely while performing them, that's all right. Don't wait to do these tasks until your overeating is under control, since doing them helps stop the overeating! You're not repudiating old habits now, but rather building new ones. And it takes time to build new habits. The changes being ushered into your life with these lessons will take a while to trickle down from your intellect to your nervous system, and developing patience is part of the process.

Impatience is nothing but the fear-mind trying to convince you it's hopeless and therefore you shouldn't even try. It's also the voice that tells you to eat the next bite before you've even finished chewing the last one, so remember that that voice is not your friend. *You* must be your friend now. And a friend is kind, so despite whatever self-disgust you feel, it is important that you be kind to yourself. This isn't a course in self-discipline, but in many ways it is a course in self-love.

You've turned unhealthy eating into a ritual, a kind of magical and secret ceremony in which you've looked to the darkness for what darkness cannot provide. You will learn to build a new ritual now: the ritual of healthy, wise, nonsecretive, and loving eating.

It all begins with a beautiful napkin.

Now in addition to thinking that's the dumbest thing you've ever heard, you might also be thinking that you already have plenty of napkins, thank you, and you do not need another one! Your drawers might be brimming with napkins—you might have inherited linen from your grandmother or bought an embroidered set from Italy or France. None of that matters now; you need a new one. *For the ones you have belong to the old you.*

It serves you at this point to understand the power of ritual. This course is asking a lot of you . . . from making lists, to writing out feelings, to procuring new items, to doing ceremony, and so forth. It is very much a *to-do* kind of book. Yet these actions are not gratuitous; they form a specific curriculum in fundamentally altering your mental habit patterns—thought-forms that have had you forever looping back to very self-destructive behavior.

It does not matter how quickly you move through these lessons, but it does matter how specifically and thoroughly you do them. You are giving a tremendous gift to yourself—even when you can't help thinking, *Oh come on, I have to do that?*—if you simply do the lessons as they are described. If they don't work, then they don't work. But if they do work, your life will change forever.

A new napkin is important; you can't build new rituals using tools that represent the old. And the last person in the world who should be discounting the power of ritual is someone who regularly performs the rituals of secret and excessive eating: driving around in the middle of the night aroused by the thought of food the way a heroin addict is aroused by the thought of heroin; opening and closing the refrigerator a hundred times in order to check whether Mommy's love might be in there now; and scanning supermarkets for hours in a heightened emotional state just looking at all the food, whether or not you're going to buy anything. No, don't try arguing that *you're not into ritual*. Nor should you discount the notion of brain triggers, when it clearly doesn't take too much of a stress factor to send you straight into the arms of food most likely to give you a temporary high and then long-term despair.

You will undermine your negative rituals by replacing them with sacred ones. These will naturally lead to healthy eating, which will naturally lead to weight loss. Amen.

Back to the napkin. It must be beautiful, as beauty is Divine. And this needn't cost you much money; you can buy a beautiful napkin for very little, definitely less than you would spend on your next binge. Choose any color and any style. Just make sure it's something you love.

Next you're going to buy a plate, and no, once again, the plates you already have will not do. Just as Orthodox Jews

have a different set of dishes for Sabbath and holiday din-
ners—meals consecrated by God—so you are going to obtain
a sacred plate for use during this process. You are rehabilitat-
ing your food appetites by making them holy.

I know you might feel that your relationship with food
is so dysfunctional . . . that your addictive patterns are so
ingrained and have gone on for so long . . . that there's simply no way to turn things around at this point. Once again,
if you had only yourself to rely on in order to make these
changes, then your anxiety would be justified.

You are not alone, however. You have placed your problem in Divine hands, and Divine power is transforming you.
That is why you are turning every step of your rebuilding
process into a sacred experience. You're taking every step
with God in mind.

You will interrupt old patterns by replacing them with
something beautiful and good. For where there is light, darkness cannot be. Where there is a connection to the sacred,
compulsion cannot stand. In the presence of the real you, all
that is not you will simply fall away.

The elements that make up this lesson are these:

- One new, beautiful napkin

- One new, beautiful glass

- One or two new, beautiful plates

- One new, beautiful knife

- One new, beautiful fork

- One new, beautiful spoon

- One new, beautiful place mat

- Two candlesticks (they can be ones you
  already have)

- Two new, beautiful candles

- One beautiful piece of music, especially wonderful to play while dining

Your family members, friends, or whoever you might live with are not being left out of this exercise, and you might wish to tell them that. The act of dedicating a single place setting is simply a response to the demands of your own healing, and not anything you're doing to separate yourself from others.

What is not allowed here are paper napkins; a paper or rubber place mat; paper or plastic plates; or a plastic knife, fork, or spoon. All of those suggest eating on the run, and one of the patterns we're moving away from is quick eating. Quick eating is a dangerous trigger for the compulsive over-eater. It triggers more quick eating, and quick eating means more food. Quick eating is a way of triggering a chemical rush and achieving an addictive high. It is very important, in laying the foundation for the new you, to cultivate a slower life. For by slowing down certain aspects of your life, you'll become a slower eater. And by eating more slowly, you are more likely to eat well.

A friend of mine told me about a dinner party she once attended in Los Angeles, along with a woman who was eating so quickly that she could hardly stuff the food in her mouth fast enough. Referring to a city about an hour outside L.A., a man at the table whispered to my friend, "She's eating like Hitler's in Pomona."

There are many reasons, certainly, for why you might eat like an army is chasing you. Maybe you feel guilty about eating whatever you're eating and want to get it over with fast so no one sees you. Maybe you have so much despair associated with eating anything that you eat quickly in an effort to eat the despair. Maybe as a child you had to eat quickly simply in order to get enough food.

It doesn't matter the reason. Sacred ritual moves molecules, transforming energy in both your mind and body. A beautiful napkin, a beautiful plate, a beautiful glass, a beautiful knife, a beautiful fork, a beautiful spoon, and a beautiful place mat will *help* you. Candles will help. And they are not immediately going into your kitchen or even into your dining room. They are going onto your altar, until you are ready to inhabit the energy they represent.

You will place everything on your altar in a beautiful array, as you prepare a feast for the real you . . . the eater who has not quite arrived yet, but is being beckoned as you read this. The you whose appetite is elegantly aligned with the spirit within you. And part of how we beckon her is by laying out her table setting and placing it on the altar.

To paraphrase a well-known adage, set the table and she will come.

Reflection and Prayer

Closing your eyes, see your altar and the table setting you have placed upon it. Now see with your inner eye a vision of an angel arriving and sitting before your new table setting. To witness the beauty, to enjoy the experience, to bless what is happening, to merely be. Allow yourself to witness this for as long as you can.

Perhaps the Divine being will invite you to sit as well, or perhaps you will find yourself merely witnessing what is happening. Whatever you see, simply allow the images to live within you.

Dear God,
Please help me begin anew,
to rebuild my temple
and restore my body.
May I learn to eat well.
Please send angels to help me.
May angels oversee my food and sit with me while I eat.
May food,
which I have so used to hurt me,
now become a blessing
and a blessing only
in my life.
Amen

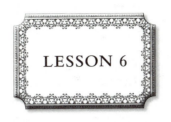

BUILD A RELATIONSHIP WITH GOOD FOOD

When my daughter was a little girl, she had a very distinct way of entering into social situations. If we went to a party or to a new school or playground, she would stand very close to me, tightly hugging my leg and not letting go. At the same time, she was intently observing the other children, watching them closely as they went about their activities.

When she felt she had seen what she needed to see, having absorbed whatever information she needed in order to feel secure in joining in, she would let go of my leg and enter easily into socializing with the other girls and boys. There was no point in saying, "Go on, honey, play with the other children!" as soon as we arrived, because she wouldn't. Yet there was never a need to coax her either, because she would get there in her own time. She simply had her process. She needed to see what was going on and sort of feel her way into a situation. Then, when she was ready, she would go.

I developed a great respect for my daughter's way of empowering herself inwardly before moving into such situations. I saw how well it worked for her. She had a child's way of simply knowing what her needs were and honoring them naturally.

In this lesson, we are honoring your need to both develop better eating habits *and* move toward them naturally, gradually, and on your own terms.

As mentioned before, there is no need to wait until you're doing well on a diet, losing weight, or even enthusiastic about any of the lessons in this course before doing them. They are meant to be your companion when you're eating well, and your companion if and when you're slipping. Whether you're feeling good or feeling despair, just keep on going.

The last lesson introduced you to the thought that you're beginning a love affair with good food. But the natural pattern of any love affair is that the initial high begins to wear off; the real-life, day-in, day-out nature of relationships begins to settle in, and your mind is tempted to distraction by something with more pizzazz. Like, say, a pizza or chocolate cake after all that salad . . . or a bagel instead of another bloody apple. And it's okay that you feel that way; if you didn't, you would not be human.

So whether you're eating cake or eating an apple, this lesson will usher you into a real relationship with food, one in which not every day will necessarily be a dramatic one, not every meal will offer an ecstatic high, and not every pain will be assuaged. But let me remind you that the relationship with food you have now is not something that offers such comforts either . . . it just pretends to.

The daily drama of an obsessive relationship with food is not the high drama of nourishment and enjoyment, but a low, cheap, pain-filled drama. The ecstatic high of excessive and unhealthy eating is not a real high at all, but a chemically triggered, addictive act of self-destruction. Your pain is assuaged by overeating for only a very short period of time, after which it comes back exponentially. This course does not ask you to be free of compulsion, but it does ask that you try to be more honest with yourself. Be honest enough to know that while good food might seem boring right now, unhealthy or excessive food is not your friend.

Once again, that does not mean to force yourself. If you're *making* yourself stop, you're only going to start again anyway. Just open your eyes to what's actually happening, and the day will come when you will simply no longer wish to hurt yourself. You will no longer want to overeat. You will be done with that, and something new will begin.

Years ago I discovered that green grapes were helpful to me in cutting down my sugar consumption. Friends told me that while grapes are a natural substance, they still contain sugar. But there's no comparison between the poison that is refined sugar and the natural sugar in ripe green grapes.

At that time I began a love affair with grapes, which continues to this day. But I didn't one day say to myself, "That's it! No more refined sugar!" Rather, there was a gradual process by which I discovered what works for me. I would eat green grapes *along with* whatever refined sugar I was eating. If I was eating a piece of cake, I'd put some green grapes on my plate as well. I don't know why I did this. Like my daughter, I simply had a natural knowing of how best to transition myself from one state to another.

And so do you.

In time, my body began to get its sweet kick from green grapes, maybe not as kicky as from cake, but kicky enough. And after even more time, my body began to register not only the kick of cake when I ate it, but also the fog it brought to my mind, the manic state it would produce within me that was then followed by physical sluggishness. I began to not *want* to go there. My body had an innate knowing of what it really wanted, and when I gave it the chance to regulate itself, then its natural intelligence and propensity for self-care kicked in.

I wasn't taking some authoritarian attitude toward my body: "Do this! Don't do that!" Rather, I worked *with* my body, making it an ally and not an enemy in my healing. I honored my emotional need to withdraw only gradually from my dysfunctional way of eating too much refined sugar, recognizing that my attachment to it had not formed in a day and would need some time to wind down. *And* I gave myself the gift of introducing into my system more healthy food choices, like I was showing up for a new relationship. Which I was!

A doctor once said to me, "Your body doesn't *want* to be sick." And *your* body doesn't want to be fat. Just as your heart knows how to beat and your lungs know how to breathe, your body knows how to calibrate its weight to that which serves the maximal functioning of your body as a whole. But artificial substances have created within you artificial appetites. When natural substances are reintroduced to your body, then your *natural appetites* will come again to the fore. And as with anything, you must give them a chance.

So it is that this lesson entails a trip to the store, to buy one thing and one thing only. Your task is to buy a piece of fruit.

You can buy any piece of fruit you choose. But there is a ritual to be honored here, which is why it would be best—if you do not have to pick up other things on this shopping trip—that all you purchase is this one item. And it's important, if possible, that you procure the fruit yourself rather than having someone else pick it up for you. Your being involved in the entirety of the process will make the ritual more impactful.

The first thing to do when you arrive home is to wash your fruit. The second thing to do is to look at it. Simply sit down in a chair and look at it.

Have you ever really looked at a pear before? Or a pomegranate? Or an apple? Have you ever noted its specific coloring, or its shape, or its size?

I once attended a couples' seminar where the trainer made both members of a couple just *look* at the other. Neither one was allowed to say a word. The exercise had to do with *seeing* each other. And while it might seem that there is little comparison between your ability to see another human being and your ability to see a piece of fruit, there is, indeed, a connection. It doesn't matter what it is you're seeing; what matters is *that you see.* And one of the reasons wholesome food seems boring to you, one of the reasons it seems not enough to you, one of the reasons it seems less than delicious to you, is because you're not *seeing* it.

Is there anything man has created that can begin to compare with the majesty of a mountain? Is there anything man has created that can begin to compare with the beauty of a flower? Is there anything man has created that can begin to compare with the power of a river or the force of a rainstorm? Then why is it that when it comes to food, people have developed this ridiculous notion that we've somehow improved on God? That chemically processed food is somehow *preferable* to what nature has to offer?

There is perfection in nature, perfection in you, and perfection in food as nature created it. Your own perfection is invoked by nature's perfection. A walk through nature calms and restores you emotionally, and natural food calms and restores you physically.

Once again, if you're still compelled to eat chemically processed foods, then eat them. The enemy is not the food, and the enemy is not you; the enemy is your obsession to eat unhealthy food and to eat it excessively. And that's okay for now. The obsessive enemy will begin to dissolve as you learn to become more of a friend to yourself.

Going to the store and buying that one piece of fruit is a *friendly* thing to do for yourself. As you begin to really *see* the food, your relationship with it will begin to grow. And this relationship will give to you in ways that you cannot even imagine right now.

Refined, chemically processed foods can give you a temporary high—that is understood. But then, if eaten excessively, they give you discomfort, sickness, despair, embarrassment, and self-hatred. You know that, but take a moment—just a moment—to truly think about what it means. Remember that speed is your enemy, whether speed eating or speed thinking. Allow yourself to digest what it means that *unhealthy eating is destroying your life.*

Natural foods—seasonal, plant-based foods like fruits, vegetables, nuts, and whole grains—restore your body, revitalize your mind, give you energy, make you more beautiful, slow the aging process, make you happier with yourself, taste even better than the other stuff once your taste buds have been restored, and improve your relationships with others because of all of the above. Don't even worry now about saying no to what you don't want; just try to say yes— however weak and weary a yes—to what is offered to you by nature's bounty.

Thousands of years ago, hundreds of years ago—and in some places, even today—people ate the food that they themselves grew. Food was part of the natural cycle of life, not something just added on to an otherwise harried existence. There was season, proportion, and rhythm to food's presence in people's lives. And those people were not some other race of being; they were your ancestors. The imprint of such naturalness is within you, based on evolutionary imperatives created over millions of years and imbedded within your cells.

Your cells have not forgotten any of this; only you have. Animals instinctively know what to eat, and so does the real you. You're not listening to your body's wisdom when you overeat; you are *overriding* your body's wisdom when you overeat. You're listening to the chatter in your mind but not to the imperatives of your body. And as you get to know your body again, as you begin to relate to it with greater respect and honor, then your relationship to its natural support system will grow stronger as well. For that is what food is: the body's support system. It maintains health and keeps the body alive. To abuse it is to abuse your body, and to abuse your body is to abuse yourself.

As always, a connection to the sacred is the way to reweave yourself into the natural harmonies of the universe. Knowing this, now take your piece of fruit—representing all healthy food with which you wish to build a new relationship—and place it upon your altar. Dedicate it in your heart to the Divine, which both created and sustains you. Give thanks for your creation and for your sustenance, and pray to be returned to your right relationship with food.

That is all you need do. God will do the rest.

Reflection and Prayer

Closing your eyes and taking a long, deep breath, allow yourself to sink into the inner temple in your mind. There you will see your sacred altar, surrounded by beauty that is invisible to the mortal eye.

First, see the place setting that has been sitting on your altar, and now see the piece of fruit you've laid upon it. Watch as an image of the Divine—whatever image occurs to you—now appears before the fruit and blesses it. Then the being lovingly hands it to you. Having been in holy hands, the fruit is now consecrated unto all that is good and healthy and wise and sane. See yourself take the fruit, and place it in your mouth.

Allow the meditation to continue for as long as is comfortable. Listen to any other message that Divine Mind gives you. Witness both the images and the thoughts that illumine your mind as you do so.

Dear God,
Please bless the food
that sits before me.
May it be filled with Your spirit
and may it feed me with Your love.
May it nourish me
that I might help nourish others.
May I never forget those who have no food.
Dear God,
please remember them, too.
Amen

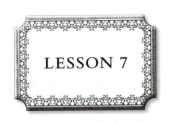

LOVE YOUR BODY

Love, and love only, produces miracles. Your primary work in doing this course is to identify where there is a lack of love in your life, and be willing to address it.

That includes your love of self, and your body is part of who you are. If you love your body when you're thin but hate it when you're not, then you love yourself conditionally, which is not love at all. If you can't love your body, you can't really love yourself.

"But how can I love my body when I hate the way it looks?" you might ask.

Begin by asking yourself: What are you hating your body *for?* For being overweight? It didn't do this to you; you did this to *it!* You haven't been abused by your body; your body has been abused by you. And yet, unlike you, it has continued to hold up its side of the relationship. It has continued to function as best it can, even though you have made it harder. It has borne excess pounds, even though it has been a burden to do so. And it has continued to support you, even though you have often failed to support *it.*

Is it your body you hate, or its size? And since all negative emotions derive from fear, if you hate your body, you must fear something. What is that? Do you fear ridicule? Or is your deeper fear—one that overrides your fear of being overweight—a fear that you'll be punished if you try to "play big" in life? Again, what are you afraid of?

Do you actually hate your body at all? Or have you simply *learned* to hate it because others hurt you so much when you were thin?

Can you remember who the first person was who envied, hated, or judged your body? Do you remember the moment you looked at your body and made a quick decision to cover it up? Was the only way to feel you "belonged" in your family to eat as excessively as your parents and siblings did? Was the only way to feel loved in your family to be as overweight as they were? Were you considered hoity-toity or stuck-up if you sought a thinner, healthier body? Was there a particular person who either looked at you strangely or said something off-color when you were a child, making you feel shame at the thought of a beautiful body? At what point did you subconsciously decide that you didn't deserve to be thin?

You can now rid yourself of the ghosts in your head. With God's help, you can forgive those who in their ignorance might have led you down a path of pain. You can now surrender your limiting beliefs. And you can renew and revitalize all aspects of yourself.

Your body has not done anything to you; it has merely reflected the raging battlefield in your mind. With this lesson, try to forgive your body for what it did not do. That is the first step in forgiving yourself for what you *did* do. It's correct to say there's been a huge misunderstanding, and the goal of this lesson is to repair and restore the relationship between you and your physical self.

When you were born, your body was perfect. Just as your spiritual self expressed itself innocently and authentically at birth, so did your physical self. Both spiritually as well as physically, the perfect imprint of your original self has not been obliterated—it has only temporarily been covered over by fear-laden thoughts. Your mind *and* your body have the ability to return to their spiritual programming when you yourself program them to do so. Your body never forgot how to be perfect; you have merely resisted its perfection.

Just as there are rituals and brain triggers that produce overeating, there are rituals and brain triggers that produce wise eating. These rituals and triggers *remind* the body of its original perfection, so it can return more easily to its perfect form and functioning.

Your relationship to food is related to millions of years of evolution, but so is your relationship to your body. There is archaeological evidence—on view at any museum exhibit of ancient artifacts—that thousands of years ago people were adorning themselves with clothes, jewelry, and other forms of decoration. The wish to appear beautiful is an ancient impulse, not some trick invented by modern advertisers to mess with your mind. Yet there is ample evidence that in various cultures throughout the ages, the idea of beauty has been vastly disparate.

For the purposes of this course, what we mean by beauty is what is beautiful to *you;* the point here is that your desire to be beautiful is a natural one, and a feeling to which you are entitled.

Maybe you've been afraid of being thin as a result of a dangerous experience in your past, and only now can you face your fear and replace it with love. In fact, being thinner does not inherently make you vulnerable to danger. Being overweight, however, does make you vulnerable . . . to embarrassment, self-hate, discomfort, ridicule, and disease.

Begin by making an apology to yourself—just a simple movement inside your heart, asking forgiveness for having mistreated such a Divine and magnificent gift as your physical body. Your body did nothing to deserve mistreatment, nor did you. But patterns of self-abuse were set into motion within you years ago, and now you must acknowledge these patterns, take full responsibility for them, atone for them, and ask God to remove these patterns so they can be cast out of your psyche. It's been a long time since you knew the experience of healthy self-love, certainly in relation to your body, and that is the miracle we pray for now.

Let's be very clear: If you are an addict, your mistreatment of your body has been extreme. It has been violent. If you have any doubt about this, stop for a moment, go into your bedroom, undress in front of a mirror, and take a good look at yourself. There you will see the scars of war: stretch marks, saggy bags of flesh produced by years of yo-yo dieting, maybe even surgical scars. Physically as well as psychologically, you've been waging war against yourself for a very long time.

But now it is time for peace. Just as with your relationship to food, your return to right relationship with your body is not something that can be fully accomplished in an instant. It would be self-defeating to expect this relationship to be fully perfected quickly after so many years of neglect. Yet the truce can begin.

Let's make a start.

This lesson involves some nice oil—even olive oil would do. Anointment by oil is a ritual used throughout the Bible, carrying a deep spiritual significance. With this lesson, you will anoint yourself with oil.

From the bottoms of your feet to the tips of your fingers, allow yourself to emotionally lean into your body, not recoil from it. In wishing to lose weight, you want your body to do something wonderful for you—and as with any relationship, it is wise to first give what you wish to receive. Give to *it*. Rub the oil into your body with acceptance, with love if you can, and with grief if necessary . . . but do not refuse it this gift. Take time over every inch of your body, paying attention to each limb, each curve, each scar, and each joint. Do not rush. Accept, affirm, apologize, and forgive.

You are learning to begin again. You are training your mind to give proper attention and respect to your body—in how you feed it, how you take care of it, how you adorn it, and how you use it. This ritual marks both the end of an abusive relationship and the beginning of an honorable one.

It would be unwise to perform this ritual in a messy bedroom or cluttered bathroom. Both mess and clutter are reflections of a distressed mind, and you deserve better from yourself. At least for now, clear up and beautify the area in which you are going to douse your body with oil. Unless you are standing in a shower, place a nice towel beneath you. Nothing with ragged edges or stains, please. You are developing the habits of beauty; the process is as important as the goal, because the goal is ultimately *inherent* in the process.

Remember that ancient kings and queens performed this ritual, and the energy they were summoning when they did so—of grace, strength, power, and beauty—is the same energy you are summoning now. Such energy is an eternal constant of the universe; it is not something that graces only a precious few, but rather an energy that is summoned by whoever summons it.

A powerful, beautiful you *is* the real you, a being of light at the center of the universe, placed there by Divine auspices and rightfully proud and dignified and joyful. No matter what the experiences of the world have done to convince you otherwise, this is a course in reclaiming truths that were always true.

Having performed this ritual, wrap yourself in a towel, and when the oil is dry, place a nice robe or other soft garment on your body. Sit quietly and allow yourself to integrate the experience of reconnecting with your body. Meditate, play music, or do anything that brings you relaxation and peace.

Now we continue. It is time to move your body.

Overweight people have often given up on movement and exercise, carrying a "What's the point?" attitude of resignation and despair. And that is understandable. But it was a former you who had those attitudes, and the old you produced a former body. Your body might still look the same, but already it is *not* the same. A new you is emerging now, and from it will emerge a new body. The real you loves to move, and so does your body when it is allowed to express itself naturally. By reconnecting to your body, you are going to learn to *listen* to your body.

Once again, don't set yourself up for failure. This lesson does not ask you to run a mile around the track or immediately go out and join a gym. Ten minutes of exercise you enjoy is better for you right now than an hour of exercise you hate. Until you can get to a place where you feel good about exercise rather than using it as an instrument of guilt, then you are not ready for more. The purpose you ascribe to something determines its effect on your life. You cannot bully yourself into a process of self-love. *Gradual* is the word here, and patient is the process.

You are simply asked to take a walk.

Walking is often underrated. It increases your metabolism and helps reconnect you to yourself. It gets your muscles moving, relaying to your body a different message than it receives when you just sit around all day. It puts you *in* your body. You've emotionally disowned your body for a long time, and it's now time to own it again.

As you walk, don't count calories. Don't obsess about how much it can or cannot do to help you lose weight. This walk is not just about your body; it's about your spirit. It's about what you're walking away from and what you're

walking toward. You are walking toward your destiny now
. . . your future, your beauty, and your happiness. It is in
itself a ritual of rebirth.

You've fed your body excessive food, perhaps, but too
little true love and care. And you will learn to change that
now. A loving approach to eating will develop more easily
when you take a more loving approach to your body in
general.

Stroll through a museum and look at paintings painted
a hundred or more years ago. Notice how people had such
beautiful bodies . . . yet they didn't belong to gyms! They
didn't exercise as a separate part of life, gritting their teeth
but doing it anyway as a way to look good. No. Adequate
movement, which itself amounts to exercise, occurred naturally as simply a part of right living. And that is what you
want it to be for you.

Exercise isn't some punishment you're going to have
to endure as a price you pay for being thin. Instead, it's an
aspect of right relationship with your body, something you
give to it in exchange for all it does for you. Your body *wants*
to move; movement helps your muscles, your heart, your
lungs, your brain. Give your body what it really wants, and
it will give to you what *you* really want.

Speaking of ancient wisdom, yoga—a Hindu practice
thousands of years old—has a near-miraculous way of reconnecting body to spirit. It is a powerful conjunction of physical and spiritual energy, and can be as gentle or as strenuous
as you make it. Yoga's simple movements make it a particularly good practice for the recovering overeater, as it begins
with basic postures that in a very easy way put you in touch
with your own body. It restores your physical functioning in
amazing ways, including your appetite for food. Whether or
not scientists have completely figured out why it works so
well, anyone who practices yoga has felt its benefits.

Once again, you don't have to sign up for a series of classes, setting yourself up to fail at something one more time! Rather, just start gently. There are links to yoga videos on the Internet, and yoga television programs abound. You don't have to begin with an hour class somewhere. Just get yourself a yoga mat. Give yourself that gift.

Watch a yoga video or DVD, and take just two minutes to try out one of the postures you see on it. Those two minutes will provide a benefit that you had not experienced yesterday. And as two turns to five, and then five turns to ten, and ten turns to a genuine desire to attend a yoga class, your body will awaken to the remembrance that it is part of a perfect universe.

Your relationship to your body has been damaged, and there is no pretending that it has not been. Like an estranged couple, you are now seeking to reunite your inner and outer selves. And in the process—as you rebuild your relationship with your body—you will reawaken to how supportive of you it really is, how powerful it really is, and how lovely it really is. It will take more than a day to achieve the kind of sweet and delightful relationship with your body to which you are entitled, but you have begun. As with any relationship, now you must feed it. Not just with healthy food—but with kindness. And movement. And love.

Place your bottle of oil on your altar as a sign of your anointment—anointment of both body and soul.

Reflection and Prayer

With your eyes closed, ask Divine Mind to guide you. See your body—exactly as it is—walking toward you. Notice your reactions to it, and where there is not love, see love begin to flow. Allow a mystical process of love and forgiveness to occur, as your soul begins to inhabit your body in a whole new way. Allow your spirit to infuse your body, and witness now as your body begins to reshape itself. See an elixir of golden light pouring over your entire body. Feel the miracle of this new beginning. Breathe in and out deeply, and surrender all.

Dear God,
May I forgive my body,
and may my body forgive me.
Repair my relationship
to this container of my soul.
Forgive me for abusing it.
Restore my mind to sanity
and my body to its proper shape.
Miraculously heal me,
dear God.
I cannot do this by myself.
Amen

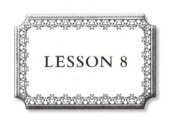

SURRENDER TO THE DIVINE

Try to surrender to the Divine not just in order to lose weight, but in order to heal your mind. Although losing weight is your primary goal, the monkey has to get off your back before the pounds will fall off your hips. An out-of-control appetite for food originates in your mind, not your body. While your mind is grasping hysterically for food, your stomach is often moaning, "Please, no more."

Almost everyone feels overstimulated at times . . . pressured . . . anxious . . . frightened of something. Different people have different ways of dealing with this anxiety, some of which are healthy and some of which are not. As an overeater, you obviously eat excessively as a way of trying to calm the anxiety monster. You use food to achieve calm, yet the calm you achieve by overeating is a temporary calm at best. The chemical reaction that goes off in your brain when you eat that cake or bread or whatever is no different from the hit a drug addict receives when the needle pierces the vein. Your anxiety will always come back in full force, both through physical stress and feelings of guilt.

Your overeating is like a roller coaster in a horror house:

1. *Anxiety:* "I'm anxious about my job [marriage, debt, or what have you]."

2. *Effort to achieve calm:* "I'll eat this bag of chips."

3. *Anxiety:* "I can't believe I just ate those chips."

At this point, you've doubled your anxiety: you have the same situational stress, *plus* the stress of having just fallen off the food wagon.

4. *Effort to achieve calm:* "I wonder what else there is to eat around here."

5. *Anxiety:* "I feel so sick. And so screwed up. I hate myself."

And the roller coaster continues. . . .

The only way to break this cycle is to deconstruct it. The only way to truly tame your anxiety is to dissolve it. The only way to calm your hysteria is to reach beyond it to the source of inner peace. And the only force powerful enough to take you there and keep you there is Divine Mind.

Many people call on God once a disaster has struck, yet the smart thing to do is to call on Him even *before* a disaster strikes. Don't just pray once your car has landed in a ditch; pray before you leave your driveway. Divine Mind is not just your comforter after a problem occurs, but also a preventive measure that helps keep problems at bay. Your task is to align your mortal mind with Divine Mind, as fear can attach itself to the mortal but not to the Divine.

When you call on Divine Mind, you're not calling on a power outside yourself. You're calling on a power that dwells within you. Spirit is a perfection that lies within all things, both protecting against chaos and reasserting harmony when chaos has happened.

Spirit makes your weight perfect because it makes *everything* perfect. Your weight is one of many areas of your life that will fall into Divine right order as you begin to give all things Divine more attention and care.

You can't get rid of your compulsion, but Spirit can. And most important of all: once you ask it to, it will. It will remove your dysfunctional hunger by feeding you what you really want.

What do you really hunger *for?*

Each day for three days, write this in your journal pages, 30 times in the morning and 30 times at night:

Dear God, please feed my hunger and restore my right mind.
Dear God, please feed my hunger and restore my right mind.
Dear God, please feed my hunger and restore my right mind.
Dear God, please feed my hunger and restore my right mind.
Dear God, please feed my hunger and restore my right mind.
Dear God, please feed my hunger and restore my right mind.
Dear God, please feed my hunger and restore my right mind.
Dear God, please feed my hunger and restore my right mind.
Dear God, Please feed my hunger and restore my right mind.
Dear God, please feed my hunger and restore my right mind.
Dear God, please feed my hunger and restore my right mind.
Dear God, please feed my hunger and restore my right mind.
Dear God, please feed my hunger and restore my right mind.
Dear God, please feed my hunger and restore my right mind.
Dear God, please feed my hunger and restore my right mind.
Dear God, please feed my hunger and restore my right mind.
Dear God, please feed my hunger and restore my right mind.
Dear God, please feed my hunger and restore my right mind.
Dear God, please feed my hunger and restore my right mind.
Dear God, please feed my hunger and restore my right mind.

Dear God, please feed my hunger and restore my right mind.
Dear God, please feed my hunger and restore my right mind.
Dear God, please feed my hunger and restore my right mind.
Dear God, please feed my hunger and restore my right mind.
Dear God, please feed my hunger and restore my right mind.
Dear God, please feed my hunger and restore my right mind.
Dear God, please feed my hunger and restore my right mind.
Dear God, please feed my hunger and restore my right mind.
Dear God, please feed my hunger and restore my right mind.
Dear God, please feed my hunger and restore my right mind.

Write this in your own handwriting rather than electronically. It is important that you try to write the sentence a full 30 times every morning and every evening, as the combination of writing and praying will have a significant impact on your psyche.

By saying this prayer, you're not asking God to take away your desire for food, and you're certainly not asking Him to take away your hunger. What you are asking is that He take away your craving—whether it's an obsessive craving or a less obvious, more gentle yet ever-present sense of "gotta have it"—so that the monkey you carry around on your back will get off and stay off forever.

You might have built many dams to keep the water of your craving from flooding your psyche and wreaking havoc on your internal landscape. Yet always, ultimately, the dam would break and the water would come rushing in. Now we are asking God to reroute the water. To send it away and send it away forever.

Whatever you eat during the day, exercise the power of prayer by saying inwardly to yourself, *Dear God, please feed my hunger and restore my right mind.*

Whether you're eating celery or you're eating cookies, *just say the prayer.* Whether you think this is powerful or you think it's hogwash, *just say the prayer*. Whether you've been doing this with every bite all day or have only now remembered to do it, *just say the prayer*.

Even if you're eating an entire cake, you can still pray while you're eating. See in your mind's eye an angel sitting with you. The angel is not there to judge you but to help you. The prayer might not bring an immediate halt to your craving, that is true. But it will begin the dismantling process.

One antibiotic pill doesn't knock out your infection on the first day, either—you have to take the whole round of antibiotics. If you have an infection, you don't say after taking one pill, "I still have a cough, so obviously this isn't working." Prayer is spiritual medicine. It boosts your spiritual immune system by increasing the depth of your surrender. Whether or not you believe it works is irrelevant. It doesn't matter what you think about surrendering to the Divine. All that matters is that you surrender.

Overeating is a battle you wage against yourself; Spirit is the power that *saves* you from yourself. It is a tincture of hope. When your mind is surrendered to the Source of all good, dysfunctional forces cannot stand for long. Like physical exercise, spiritual exercise works if you do it. Surrendering to the Divine is an issue of mental discipline, in which you train yourself to put God first. This is not difficult; it is simply different. In all things, spiritual surrender marks the end of struggle and the beginning of true ease.

In the moment when you are dealing with a compulsive urge, even the deepest religious faith can be rendered ineffective by the power of addiction. With this lesson, you learn to cultivate the mental discipline of calling on God as a regular practice. Don't call on Divine Mind to help you only in the hour of your need, but rather call on it as a way to cultivate and maintain serenity. This lesson will help dismantle your resistance to doing that. It empowers you to reach beyond your hysteria and ultimately dissolve it, by reestablishing your connection to the source of inner peace.

In the moments when you are *not* surrendered to love, you are bound by fear. When you are not consciously and proactively calling down the light, you are vulnerable to darkness. And it is light, not darkness, for which your spirit yearns. Spiritually, you want to lose weight not just to become less flesh, but to become *more spirit*. Every moment when you eat inappropriately is simply a moment when you are starving for Spirit's love, can't find it where it actually exists, and therefore struggle to find it elsewhere.

You are learning to look into the eyes of fear and stare it down. To reach for Spirit and feel it reach back. To pray for a healing of your mind and to experience your deliverance. You are waking up to your spiritual power.

One day you will walk up to the refrigerator, open the door, and find yourself only looking for what's good for you. It will dawn on you that you are behaving, without even thinking about it, along a new line. You are searching for healthy and appropriate food, and nothing else. There has been a pattern interruption, something you didn't consciously make happen through an act of will. It represents a new synapse, a new pattern emerging, and thus new hope. You did your part, and God did His.

But you cannot ask for Divine help in one area of your life without being willing to surrender *every* area of your life. You can't just surrender food; you must try to surrender every thought and feeling. For every thought and feeling contributes either to your disease or to its healing.

Spiritual surrender is a full-throttle willingness to let go of everything—every thought, every pattern, and every desire—that blocks love from entering into you and extending through you. If you're unkind, that blocks your healing.

If you withhold forgiveness, that blocks your healing. If you're dishonest, that blocks your healing. Every issue in your life is related somehow to your struggle with food. Nothing is separate from who you are and what you're manifesting. And that's what makes this issue in your life an invitation to become your most beautiful self—not only on the outside, but on the inside, too.

Remember to place your journal back on your altar when you are done. This will uplift the energy of your prayers.

Reflection and Prayer

As you did in Lesson 3, close your eyes and see your body infused with light. Once again, every cell is filled with an elixir poured forth from Divine Mind. Spirit surrounds you as you release yourself fully into the arms of love.

Hold this image for at least five minutes. Breathe out your burdens and breathe in the light. See it pour into your body and extend outward from your flesh until you are bathed all around in a golden glow. Continue this visualization for as long as it feels comfortable to do so.

Continue with whatever food plan works for you. But whatever and whenever you eat, surrender the experience to Spirit. There is no way to fail here. Whatever you eat, see it as a Divine experience, and in time the experience will be transmuted. The point now is not what you eat or don't eat, or whether you exercise or do not exercise. The point is to turn your relationship with your body, with food, with exercise—with everything—into a spiritual experience.

Dear God,
I know You know
that I need repair.
I am so removed
from the wisdom of my body
and the love in my heart
when it comes to food.
I am overwhelmed by the thought
of healing myself,
and so I pray, dear God,
that You will do this for me.
Change my thoughts,
heal my cells,
repair my appetites,
restore my body.
Such praise I give,
and thanks, dear God.
Amen

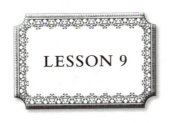

INHABIT
YOUR BODY

I don't remember, when I was very young, either hating my body *or* loving it. I simply remember inhabiting it with a child's natural innocence and enjoyment. As a little girl, I remember joyfully parading around my house in ruffled underwear. I remember wearing a bikini—we called it a "two-piece" then—and having no breasts yet to fill it out. I remember being so little (or so Texan) that we didn't call it "naked," we called it "nekked!"—and there was nothing sexual or shameful about it.

Later, however, something happened. It didn't happen for me in one traumatic moment; it happened gradually and insidiously, as it does for many people. I was never molested as a child or physically or emotionally traumatized by a specific event. But an accumulation of toxic moments became an oceanic wave of anxiety that permeated my mind and turned my body into a point of confusion.

For reasons that remained buried within my subconscious for a very long time, I came to emotionally disown my body. Twisted thought-forms came into my mind via so

111

many sources, both personal and cultural, that the only way I knew how to cope with them was to disown the part of me they referred to. What had once been a thing of pleasure became a painful subject. I simply dissociated from what I couldn't figure out. My body became like a house I no longer lived in.

For some people, dissociation from a natural and healthy sense of their body occurs as a result of a traumatic event or experience. For others, adolescence itself is traumatic. It ultimately doesn't matter so much *how* the trauma occurred, as much as that you repair the gaping wound it left within you. Whatever is broken in your body began with broken-ness in your heart. Being an overeater, the chances are very good that the history of your relationship with your body is complicated, but with this lesson, you will identify your wounds in order to best address your pain.

The criminality of rape, molestation, and so forth—as well as our need to protect against such transgressions as a society—has been well established. But the lesser assault of toxic thought-forms can lead to serious consequences as well. Whether your personal history involves sudden trauma or gradual trauma, your task is to understand it so it can be healed.

As an example, on the next several pages I have listed the personal history that led to my own dissociation from my body. Your list will be in some ways different from and per-haps in some ways similar to mine. One thing most of us do share is a psychological crisis that came to a head around the age of puberty. Thoughts of innocence turned to thoughts of pain, and that which was healthy began to be sick.

Sick Thought #1: *My body isn't good enough.*

I read *Seventeen* magazine, so I knew this for sure. So many girls were curvier, taller, sexier, and so forth. Karen had bigger breasts, Trudie had better hair, and Cheryl just had that *thing* that boys wanted.

Conscious: My body is ugly. It isn't good enough.

Subconscious: My body deserves to be punished.

Sick Thought #2: *My body makes grown-ups squirm, so there must be something wrong with it.*

I had no idea why my seventh-grade English teacher, who had seemed to adore me, got so weird around me once my body began to develop. I had the vague feeling that her strange attitude had something to do with my body and my budding sexuality, but there was no one and nothing to guide me through the vagaries and land mines of puberty.

I went back to speak to this teacher when I was in my early 30s, to confront her about what I had experienced and to ask her if I had simply imagined it. She said to me—and the day would come when I understood this—that I had no idea what it meant to be a woman watching her own sexuality fade while young girls around her were beginning to blossom into theirs.

My teacher had not meant to hurt me; she had not consciously rejected me; she had simply felt a natural disappointment—disappointment she did not know how to process except by projecting it onto others—in relation to a situation that had nothing to do with my life and everything to do with hers.

I also remember my music teacher staring at my breasts once during a piano lesson. This was before there was the social consciousness about these things that there is today. He only stared, but if you're sitting at the piano and a young girl is standing next to you, you're staring from up close.

How I wish I could reach back in time and give that man a piece of my mind. He died before I had a chance, but if I

A COURSE IN WEIGHT LOSS

could have, I would have paid him a visit along the same line as the one I paid to my seventh-grade English teacher.

Conscious: Grown-ups act strangely around me now that my body has changed.

Subconscious: My body must be bad.

Sick Thought #3: *Daddy doesn't want to be around me as much anymore.*

My father's attitudes about sex and sexuality—while certainly not prudish when it came to my mother!—were somewhat old-fashioned. He seemed to want his daughters dressed in pink lace and white gloves long past the time when our age or the fashion of the times called for either one. He seemed somewhat uncomfortable with my budding sexuality, yet I had no idea what that meant or what to do with it. How could I?

I remember a moment—I think many women have such memories—when I went to sit on Daddy's lap and he made me get up and sit somewhere else. This was a small but emotionally devastating moment for me, although I realize now that it represented what would be a reasonable act on the part of fathers when their no-longer-little girls come to sit on their laps. All I could possibly have known then was that once I passed puberty, my father began to look at me in a different way. I didn't feel like I was *okay* in his eyes anymore, as though somehow I embarrassed him.

My father continued to want to take me to the zoo on Sundays, long past the time when going to the zoo was my idea of a really cool Sunday outing. The only way he knew how to relate to me, it seemed, was if I remained a little girl.

The inability of my parents to help me transition—and make their own, as well—through my archetypal maidenhood was a product not of their lack of love for me, but of their psychological ignorance regarding how to handle the experience. There is nothing to forgive here; there are simply things to understand.

Conscious: Daddy doesn't treat me like he used to.

Subconscious: Who I am now sends Daddy away. My new body is a bad thing.

Now just around the time when Daddy didn't seem to want to be around my new body, some younger males did. And since I was bereft at what seemed to be the loss of my father's love, I was subconsciously looking around to replace it. Add to that the so-called sexual liberation of the 1960s, and I see myself now as having been doomed to some serious confusion and self-destructive behavior. Like millions of others, I went looking for love in too many places, almost ensuring that I would find it too few times.

Yet many of my experiences were positive. There is one moment deeply ingrained in my memory that is a precious part of my past.

I was walking through Hermann Park in Houston on a beautiful late afternoon. I was wearing a long culottes outfit, red with white polka dots, which I can see in my mind as though I had worn it yesterday. I was probably 16 years old. A young man around the same age as I was walked by, and he looked at me in an innocent and appropriate, yet decidedly male, way.

I had never experienced such a moment before. My body had a sexual charge now, and he was old enough to notice it. He was no longer a little boy, and I was no longer a little girl. But the energy was wonderful, neither lascivious nor predatory, and our momentary encounter has remained within me as one of my most treasured memories. We didn't even speak, but in that moment, I felt for the first time that I was a woman and not a little girl.

That experience in the park was a lovely thing, like an enchanted image from a fairy tale. But it was not the reality of ordinary, day-to-day life. I didn't even meet the young man. The value of the experience was that it gave me a window into the innocent, ideal beauty of my own untainted sensuality. Life would provide me with positive experiences of my own physicality. But the purpose of this inventory is not just to celebrate the good; it is also a way to root out the bad, by seeing it, understanding it, and forgiving it.

Sick Thought #4: *My body is what attracts love.*

I know now that my body does not attract love; *I* do. My body attracts *attention,* but it does not necessarily attract love. It is my spirit and not my body that both magnetizes and holds on to love.

We are living in a society that gives to sexual chemistry a role beyond what it actually has in the greater scheme of things, and all of us have been privy to this dangerous confusion. Sexual chemistry is important, obviously, because without it the human race wouldn't continue. But the idea that if *I am sexy enough, he will love me* is a tragic error in thinking. If I am sexy enough he might *want* me, that is true, but whether he loves me or not is based on way, way more than what happens in bed.

It's odd to consider now, but much of the sexual "liberation" of the '60s was not true liberation for women at all. We were liberated to *have* sex, but we were still doing it primarily as a way to please men. We weren't yet aware—nor were most men at the time—that our true value lay in something much more important than our sexuality. That began to fundamentally change in the '70s, not the '60s.

Conscious: Sex is fun.

Subconscious: If I do this enough, I will be loved.

Sick Thought #5: *My value lies not in my body at all. I am only valuable because of my mind.*

When the correction came, it went way overboard. The dangerous thought that a woman's body was all that made her attractive was replaced by the equally dangerous thought that her *mind* was all that made her attractive. Millions of us bought into the notion that sexual attractiveness merely played into male chauvinistic fantasies that reduced women to sex objects. It's about then that we thought it was cool to burn our bras, to stop shaving our legs or armpits, to refuse to let men open doors for us . . . but then to go at it like bunnies at the end of the day, of course.

Knowing that our value lay in much more than just the look of our bodies was a huge realization. But the fact that a woman's body isn't the essence of her value does not mean that her body has no value!

Thinking, as many of us did in those days, that any male celebration of our looks was traitorous to some feminist ideal—while we sure were enjoying all that celebration once the lights were down—inevitably created a psychic ambivalence and dissociation. On the one hand, we were young enough to enjoy the amazing sensations of youthful sexuality. At the same time, we thought the only way to be really cool was to deny its importance.

Conscious: My sexuality isn't what is important about me.
Subconscious: My body isn't important.

It was at about that time that my compulsive eating began. Added to the above was the loneliness of my college years, during which time I added the "freshman 15" pounds that such experience often entails. By then I was pretty much off and running straight into the darkness of food hell, where I remained for almost a decade.

A Course in Miracles teaches us to beware the power of an unrecognized belief. I have come to understand that based on my own personal history, I had an unrecognized belief that my body was not good, was not lovable, was not even important . . . and then I set out, unconsciously, to prove myself right.

Dissociation from the body, for whatever reason, robs you not just of the joy of healthy eating, but of even identifying with your own body. Dissociation is when you see yourself here, and your body is *there*. It's a sense that you are somehow separate from your body, which is a tragic split from self.

I am well aware that the gradual trauma of my own body history is nothing compared to what many others have experienced. For those who have suffered physical abuse—sexual or otherwise—an overwhelming horror has elicited an overwhelming need to escape from pain at whatever cost.

Many overeaters don't actually inhabit their body so much as hover above it or to the side of it some 6 to 12 inches, reenacting an ancient response—tragically necessary at one time—to a shattering experience such as being whipped or raped. This experience might go back to the earliest days of childhood, even as far back as three or five years old.

According to a study at the University of Pennsylvania School of Medicine, up to 33 percent of American girls are molested, and research tracking the connection between a history of molestation to obesity is in its early stages.

For many people, an instinctive escape mechanism that developed originally in response to such abuse now trips like a switch in reaction to almost any form of stress. The subconscious commanded, "Flee! Flee!" and the child who was powerless to flee physically developed the capacity to flee psychologically.

For the adult that the child one day becomes, the command to "Flee!" still exists not only in reaction to danger, but also in reaction to almost any form of physical or emotional discomfort. This applies painfully, and perhaps particularly, as a reaction to sexual intimacy.

Healthy sex requires that you truly inhabit your body, and for a victim of sexual abuse, this would feel like surrendering to a warning bell. If at a moment of profound trauma your spirit left your body to escape the reality of the experience, and never fully reentered it on a consistent basis, then how do you escape your escapism in order to show up for sex? This could obviously be very difficult.

Overeating becomes, for those dissociated from their body for whatever reason, a way to reenact the original escape from pain and confusion. In one moment of chemically induced numbness, you can feel, "Ah, I escaped . . ." Reenacting your earlier escape from physical trauma, you once again leave the realm of your suffering behind . . . if even for a moment. *A Course in Miracles* teaches that you create what you defend against. Defending against a physical trauma, you've created a new one: the trauma of overeating.

Today's lesson begins to unravel this route of horror, the instinctive path you still walk in an effort to deal with pain and stress. These days, your stress might look nothing at all like the physical abuse you endured as a child—it might be something as mundane as your need to pick the kids up at school, get them to soccer on time, and still get to the dry cleaners before they close—yet your subconscious mind continues to interpret your stress as danger and reacts to it that way. "I must get out of here!" is all you know. And you "escape" into food.

Your assignment now is to write your own personal story—where things went right and where things went wrong. Explore how you came to dissociate from, fear, and perhaps even hate, your body. And don't expect all of this to be easy. Some of it might be funny, some of it might be horrifying, some of it might be ridiculous, and some of it might be extremely painful. What is important is that it be honest and true.

By writing down your history, you will come to understand it more fully. And by understanding it more fully, you will emerge from the darkness of your subconscious bondage to fears that were born in a distant past. These fears can be dissolved today, through grace and through love. In doing this lesson, you begin the process.

Use your journal pages to write your story, giving full attention to both good and bad memories. Return this book to your altar after every entry you write.

Reflection and Prayer

Close your eyes and relax into a meditative state. During this time, allow your mind to return to your experience of yourself as a baby, then a toddler, then a small child, and so on.

During every phase of the meditation, allow yourself to see what you looked like at a certain time in your life, how you felt about your body, what you went through, who was involved, where things went well, where you were hurt, where you went unconscious, where you dissociated from your body, where you began to hate your body, what attitudes you formed about sex, where you decided to cover up your body with fat, and so forth. You will come to realize that your issues with eating have ultimately little to do with food, and everything to do with thoughts about yourself.

This will not be a quick meditation, or a casual one. There are many feelings from your past that have remained unprocessed . . . many experiences that you have not yet looked at through the lens of time and forgiveness . . . and many people, including yourself, whom you have failed to understand. Use this course as a path to understanding now what you could never have understood before.

Dear God,
I give to You my past
and ask that You explain it to me.
Unravel, dear God,
the cords of confusion
that bind me.
Free me from the bondage
of blindness and misunderstanding.
Return me, dear God,
to a sense of my body
that is Your truth, and no one else's,
that is sacred and not impure,
that is loving and not punishing,
that is joyful and not painful,
that is healthy and not diseased.
Please, dear God,
undo my past and return me to my
innocent self.
Amen

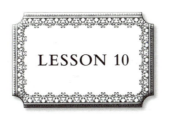

CONSECRATE YOUR BODY

Your body is not separate from your mind so much as it is a reflection of it. As you change your mind, you change every cell in your body.

Such thoughts as *I am fat, I am ugly,* and *I hate my body* are like commands given to your body to materialize accordingly. If you think negatively about your body, your body will reflect your negativity. If you think lovingly about your body, then your body will reflect your love. And there is no such thing as a neutral thought. What is not love, is an attack. And what *is* love, is a miracle.

Let us now consecrate your body to be used for holy purposes. Holy purposes are love and love only, and as you consecrate your body to love, all that is not love can no longer hold sway within it. Whatever is dedicated to the purposes of love is protected from the energy of chaos.

Write down this line: *I eat in a way that supports my being of service to love.*

That is a good one, by the way, to put on a Post-it and keep on your refrigerator door.

With this lesson, embrace a new perception of your body in order to make manifest a new physical reality.

Begin each day with a prayer:

Dear God,
As I awaken on this day,
may my body and mind serve Your purposes.
May nothing but Your Spirit
be upon me.
May my body be a temple to Your Spirit
and a conduit of love.
Amen

As you head to the kitchen, the voices of both fear and love will be bubbling up within you. Fear would have you eat an unhealthy breakfast, full of refined carbohydrates and sugar and such foodstuffs as that. Or not eat breakfast at all. That way you will have a harder time feeling the lightness of your spirit, and fear's purposes will thus be accomplished. But what would you eat if the only purpose of your body today was to serve love's purposes? Would you not eat a light, healthy breakfast in order to support your body in doing God's work?

Begin today to change your body by thinking of it as a temple for your soul. Your body is like an infinitely precious suit of clothes. It is not essentially who you are, but it can be a sacred container for your spirit.

Things of this world are holy or unholy depending on the purpose that the mind ascribes to them; the holy purpose of your body is to serve your loving communion with life itself. That is what it means to consecrate your body. To honor your body, to treat it well, to add to its care and protection from harm, is to honor the Divine by honoring your body's spiritual mission. The holy purpose of *anything* you do in the world is to honor the Divine, and your body is the physical basis for everything you do.

In a previous lesson, you began to take stock of psychological assaults to which your body has been exposed throughout your life. With this lesson, you will begin to shift your body identification from that of a damaged thing to that of a holy thing. Both your mind and your body will go through a spiritual initiation, transforming first the one and then the other. The mind will shift, and the body will follow.

Your body was not created to house your fears, but rather to house your love. And in your heart, you know this. Your deepest yearning is not just for your body to look good but also for your body to *be* good. With this lesson, you will take your wish that this were so, turn it into an intention that it be so, expand that into a willingness that it be so, invite Divine Mind to help you make it be so . . . and it shall be so.

Your task now is to consecrate your body, not just as a general intention but rather as an actual directive from your conscious to your subconscious mind. You will write down your loving intentions in order to contain and harness their power.

In the last lesson, you wrote about your past; in this one, you will write about your present. In any moment or any hour in which your body is dedicated to the purposes of love, it is less prone to the purposes of fear.

Let's begin with what might be a typical day. Write down the following categories:

1. Waking up

2. Breakfast

3. Morning activities

4. Lunch

5. Afternoon activities

6. Dinner

7. Evening hours

Now write two versions of this list.

First, write down what you do now. Be honest with yourself; no one else needs to read this. Go through your day and write down everything you do. Describe a typical day in your life: write down what you eat, what you do with your life, how you feel about what you do, your thoughts about other people, and so forth.

If you go through this too quickly, just jotting down "I did this" or "I did that," then you will not receive the greatest value from this lesson. Your task—and the gift you are giving yourself—lies in being deeply honest about how you live now. This lesson gives you the chance to look into the mental control room of your life and observe the way you program your experience.

Next, write a second description of your day. Yet this time, consciously redesign your life. Do not just write what you're doing or how you feel about it; rather, describe your day from the perspective of your higher mind. Write about the life you *choose,* rather than one lived powerlessly at the effect of habitual emotional and behavioral patterns. Choose to be the *real you* as you write this: a conduit of God's love, here to extend love and to do love's work on Earth. Allow love to dictate both your purposes and your plans for the day.

This will not necessarily be easy—at times it might even feel foolish—because you're training your thoughts to flow in a different direction than they're used to flowing. Yet that is the point. As you create the space for love in every area of your thinking, you create a space for love in every area of your life.

Write either about the day now past or the day ahead. Below is an example of such conscious redesign:

1. Waking Up

After I wake up, I do not let too much time go by before praying. I thank God for giving me this day, and I pray that all I do today will be of service to love. I pray for my family, for my friends, for my country, and for the world. I surrender the day ahead, asking that it be blessed and that I be a blessing on it.

I offer a kind "Good morning!" to those I see. Friends or family who live with me, or any others who are in my house this morning, receive a pleasant greeting from me. With a smile, a hug, a positive word; or by giving them a glass of orange juice, I do what I can to be a loving presence in their lives.

From brushing my hair to putting on a nice robe; from making breakfast for my children to giving encouragement to my spouse; from opening up a window or door to breathe in the beauty of the new morning, I celebrate and add to the good that is all around me.

When there is quiet, I take the opportunity to read scripture or inspirational literature, to pray and meditate, to reflect and contemplate on all that is loving and Divine. I consciously surrender my day to God.

When there is time, I do something loving for my body such as light weights, yoga, or a short walk. I do this as a blessing on my body, gratefully serving it as it so serves me. Even if I don't exercise for a prolonged period, I do some kind of movement. Daily I do this . . . helping sustain my heart and lungs and other vital organs, allowing my skin to receive the nourishment of the sun, stretching my muscles to make and keep them strong . . . I am taking care of my body in order to prepare myself for joy and for better service to the world.

Note how different such programming is from what fear would pour into your mind. The thinking of Divine Mind is 180 degrees away from the thinking of the world, and it is your choice—as well as your responsibility to yourself—to cultivate the thinking that will lift you above your wounded self.

If fear rules your thinking—if your intentions are not loving but rather some form of, *Oh darn, another day just like the last one. . . . They can get their own breakfast. . . . I don't care what he does. . . . I don't care how I look. . . . I just want to eat something. . . . I don't owe anything to anyone. . . . I don't want to take time to pray. . . . I don't want to take the time to walk. . . . I hate my life. . . . What point is there to any of this? . . . There is nothing to be happy about*—then do not expect your physical appetites to do anything other than reflect the fear that is in your mind. And for you, fear has taken a specific form: the compulsion to eat inappropriately.

It might seem at times that you have no control over your urge to eat—and for all practical purposes, many times you do not. But you *always* have free will regarding what you think, and as you begin to *think* differently, in time you will begin to *eat* differently. Your compulsion will dissolve in the presence of the Divine.

2. Breakfast

I feed my body this morning with loving nourishment. I do not harm it with unhealthy food and drink; rather, I fuel it with healthy food or drink that I know will make my cells more vital.

With the food I eat, I help my body have greater energy and health, as well as be more aligned with the spirit within me. My body is a holy temple; I joyfully feed it with food that supports my Divine purpose in the world.

3. Morning Activities

My morning is spent doing things that contribute goodness and light to my family, my community, and my world. I use my body as an instrument of peace, as I seek to share peace with others. My body serves me in doing good and living joyfully.

At every moment, I breathe in the perfection of the universe and breathe out any toxicity in my mind or body. My body supports me by showing up as a positive force for everyone I encounter. My body is a temple in which my spirit resides, supporting me in extending love to all I see.

At work, I pray only to be an instrument of peace. I pray for all those with whom I work or will encounter. I pray for their happiness and well-being. I forgive quickly and try not to judge others.

I surrender my job to Spirit and ask that with my work, I serve the greater good. I feel the cells of my body awaken as I think these things; I feel my body energized as I apply it to love's purposes in the world.

While I do chores, I ask that Spirit make even mundane activities a thing of goodness. As I do my family's laundry, I think with love about the cherished ones whose clothes I am about to clean, and feel gratitude for the clothes I own. As I go to the store, I give thanks that I can afford to buy the essentials I need. As I pick up something for a family member or do a chore for someone else, I surrender any resentment I feel and ask to be filled with a lighter attitude.

I know my body is responding to every thought I think, and I choose to think with love. This way, my body is made healed and whole.

4. Lunch

As I stop to eat lunch, I thank my body for the way it has served me so far today, and commit anew to its sustenance and nourishment. I use lunch as an opportunity to nourish not only my body but also my soul. I stay away from frantic environments, and cultivate peace as I eat.

I purchase healthy food or bring it from home. I am aware that unhealthy choices abound in the world around me. I do not judge those choices, but neither do I participate in this cultural weakness by eating unhealthy food, even if it is most easily available to me. I make this choice in order to do right by my body and my mind. I realize that my body is a holy temple and deserves only nutritious, restorative food.

I silently say grace before my meal, thanking all the people who contributed to the manufacture and preparation of the food I eat, thanking the earth for giving it to me, and thanking God for the fact that I have food at all.

5. Afternoon Activities

I choose to give my body rest, that it might have a chance to recharge. I take responsibility for carving into my day even a short period of time during which my body and soul can realign with Spirit, casting off the stress of a world that is moving too fast. I allow my body some sort of afternoon movement as a way to reinvigorate itself. Even a walk around the block is good for my body and programs it in a healthy way.

I continue to give it positive affirmations of love and encouragement as I move through the rest of the day, thanking God for the miracle of my body and dedicating it continuously to the purposes of love.

Before dinner, I take time to rest, pray, meditate, do yoga, take a bath, light candles and/or incense in my room, and otherwise give my body and soul the chance to de-stress after the busyness of the day.

I value rest and recognize its importance. I know that I alone am responsible for cultivating a lifestyle that supports my health, my good, and my serenity. I know my body may react with compulsive behavior if I fail to proactively create a peaceful environment. I surround my body with peace so that it will be at peace.

6. Dinner

As I prepare for dinner, I dedicate this important time to goodness and love. I prepare myself inwardly to be a vessel of love's goodness. The goodness of my family gathered around a dinner table. The goodness of my partner coming home to a loving environment after a stressful day. The importance of my children knowing that someone is waiting to nourish and listen to them at dinnertime.

During dinner, I consciously reject the frantic stimuli of the world. I turn off the television and computers and insist that my children do so as well. I prepare a beautiful table, perhaps with candles or fresh flowers. I say grace before the meal and include my family. I take responsibility for a healthy environment while I eat, for I know that such an environment supports healthy habits.

In the food I prepare, the way I dress, the way I behave, and the way I interact with others, I pray to be a positive influence on those I love. I feed healthy food, healthy words, and healthy energy to others and myself. I see the food I eat as a way to give thanks and service to the body I have been miraculously given, and to feed those I love with gratitude and devotion.

7. Evening Hours

I am grateful for having eaten lightly enough to have energy for a productive evening. I use my time to deepen my relationships, tend to the emotional needs of my family, expand my mind, increase my participation in the world around me, and delve into the mysteries of life that emerge more clearly in the nighttime hours. If my environment supports it, I take the opportunity to walk, hopefully able to see the stars in the nighttime sky.

A cup of herbal tea is my evening companion, supporting me in pacifying my physical system as I head toward sleep. I allow my body and soul to reveal their needs to me, as I use these hours to conclude my day in a positive way. I attend to the needs of those around me, honoring my role as parent, mate, and friend.

I enjoy my life as it is. I honor its demands, and honor my desires. I take the time to breathe in the realization of how fortunate I am, and commit to living ever more fully with each passing day. I give thanks for having lived this day, and I give blessings to all the world.

It might seem at first that such a positive description is simply fiction. And if you have been living the life of an active addict, then that might be true. But as you write a different description of your life, you create a line of possibility that did not exist before. Do not underestimate the power of your mind to reprogram your experience.

Enlightened lines of thought counter dysfunctional habits. Even one moment of insight—looking around the food court at lunchtime and realizing with blazing clarity that its main offerings *are bad for you and that you can choose differently;* looking at others and realizing that the healing of your dysfunctional habits is intimately tied up with the love you extend—leads to another insight, leading at last to your escape from food hell.

It is not enough to simply read what I wrote in the last few pages. In order to receive the benefit of this lesson, you must write down a description of your own day. Begin by writing about your present life—simply describing what is— and then reading it. Allow yourself to see the gap between the fear that is, and the love that could be. Recognize how often your thought-forms are weak, fear based, and almost sure to produce dysfunction.

Now write a new statement of intention, a manifesto of love for all the things you will do during your day, and allow yourself to gently lean into it. There is nothing new for you to do, so much as something new for you to imagine. This new architecture for your life is not meant to tyrannize you, but to lead you to freedom.

A new way of eating, one that fundamentally and permanently transforms you, can only be created within the context of a new way of being. Your desire to eat differently is a sacred calling to take your entire life to a deeper level. If you don't feel it yet, that's okay. But do still write it down, for that is the first step. And, of course, return your journal to the altar when you are done.

Reflection and Prayer

Sitting quietly with your eyes closed, see your day ahead. With every action you know you will be taking, actively see how you would probably behave given past patterns. Now ask Divine Mind to reveal to you the possibilities for a more enlightened you.

See things you do; now see more loving things you *could* do, or how you could do what you do more lovingly. See yourself speaking harshly or negatively, if that is what you tend to do; now see yourself speaking gently and kindly. See yourself eating poorly or hurriedly, excessively or secretively; now see yourself eating with appropriateness and self-care.

As you allow Spirit to show you a new way of living, you will naturally see within your mind's eye a new way of eating. You will imagine what it looks like and feels like to feed your body lovingly, to allow food to be part of a larger matrix of love in your life. By imagining it, holding the vision, and allowing the vision to come alive within you, you will gradually experience it coming to pass.

> *Dear God,*
> *Please show me how to live in love.*
> *May a new kind of eating*
> *come naturally from a new way of being.*
> *I devote not only my appetites*
> *but every part of me to You.*
> *Where fear has blocked me,*
> *may love now free me.*
> *Please teach me, God,*
> *how to live my life*
> *in the light of love,*
> *that fear shall be no more.*
> *Amen*

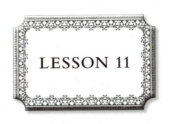

RITUALIZE THE CHANGE IN YOU

I have a girlfriend named Kathy for whom healthy eating is an art. Her example has had more of an impact on my thinking and behavior than she realizes, as I find myself, in her words, "leaning into" a more healthy diet. I don't have a goal around this so much as I am involved in a process. I realize what a gift she has been to me—someone I know whose eating is grounded in natural, nutritious, and spiritual principles.

I've been a guest in Kathy's home several times, and consequently I've been privy to what is in her refrigerator and kitchen cupboards. Her vegan world is like a mysterious universe to me. I don't make notes . . . but I do observe, and I ask questions. I'm not running out and trying to force myself to become a vegetarian, but I've deepened my understanding about connecting my spirituality to the way I eat. It's undeniable that knowing Kathy has had a subtle but powerful influence on how I think about food.

As a student of *A Course in Miracles*, I know that relationships are assignments made by a loving universe, giving everyone involved the opportunity for soul growth. Some-one who inspires you to eat in a healthier way is an important figure in your life. Kathy rarely talks to me about her passion for healthy food—part of her power, in fact, is that she doesn't seek to pressure others—but her presence is like a guiding light as I move toward a healthier diet.

This lesson involves finding your own Inspirer, as Kathy is mine. Whether your issue is excessive eating or simply better eating, there is power in having a living example to look to.

Your Inspirer is much like what 12-step programs call a sponsor. This may be someone who has healed from food compulsion and now inspires you in your own healing. This person might help you navigate the various temptations that confront you, and can understand what you're going through in ways that others never could. Or your Inspirer might be someone who has never suffered from a weight issue at all, but simply demonstrates a way of being with food and with his or her body that you can learn from. It's what your Inspirer demonstrates now, more than what he or she experienced in the past, that makes this individual a beacon of hope for you as you move forward. His or her very presence demonstrates what's possible.

Once you have identified your Inspirer, you will ask this person to participate in a personal initiation ceremony that marks the beginning of a new phase of your life. This initiation is not just a farewell to your compulsive self, but also a calling forth of the spirit of your true being. Rituals such as this have a way of grounding the holy. Once your psychological responses are infused with Spirit, you'll feel more personally capable of making real change.

The initiation ceremony is sacred, and the people you ask to participate in it with you are important. You will ask them to "stand up" for you as you make a journey into conscious weight loss.

It is conscious in that it goes beyond the mere letting go of weight; it is a letting go of the part of your personality for which eating excessively and self-destructively has felt natural. Your losing weight is not just the removal of excess weight from your body; it is the removal of unwanted dynamics from your mind.

You are building new synapses in your brain, new tracks in your nervous system, and new thought-forms in your problem-solving repertoire. This process—leaving you no longer at the mercy of your out-of-control habits, and giving you dominion over your body—makes your journey away from food compulsion a spiritual initiation.

With this lesson you create a ceremony, through which you pass from a formerly weakened to a newly strengthened you. This journey is a spiritual death and rebirth of sorts. The aspect of yourself that has struggled with weight will be disappearing, and the aspect that is free of such struggle will rise from the ethers of a more spiritualized consciousness.

By agreeing to play the role of your Inspirer, this person willingly contributes his or her goodwill and support to your effort at weight loss. Your Inspirer may never even talk to you about your struggle once your initiation ceremony is done, or he or she may listen to you unconditionally and without judgment day in and day out. Either way, that goodwill remains as a beacon of hope and a path of excellence for you to follow. Silently or verbally, this individual provides support and inspiration that will bless your path.

Enough! with looking at thinner people and feeling jealousy or a twinge of self-hate. Now that you have an Inspirer, you will begin to change your perception of those for whom weight is not a problem, and instead begin to see them as your teachers. They teach by example. Looking at them will no longer trigger pain for you, but instead bring you a sense of joyful possibility. Your Inspirer will be an example of someone whose healthy weight invites you to move toward your own.

Your Inspirer is only half of your team, however. There is someone else who is equally as important to your initiation ceremony, and that is your Permitter.

This is someone with whom you share a different and unique bond: he or she has the experience of food hell just like you. This person is either inwardly preparing for his or her own healing journey or, like you, is already involved in taking action toward conscious weight loss. The Permitter's role here is to grant you the emotional permission to break free of the cycle of compulsive eating, even if it means saying no to dysfunctional social interactions upon which you have become dependent.

The fear-based mind is very big on building alliances, but they are alliances of suffering. We often find ourselves subconsciously collaborating with others who share the same wounds we do, unconciously supporting each other in justification and denial. Alliances can be powerful networks of support and encouragement, but in the hands of the fear-mind, they are anything but that.

Perhaps your entire family is overweight and views your decision to break free of the familial pattern as some sort of traitorous act. "Who are you to think you can get thin? Who are you to start eating differently? Are you making us wrong for the way we eat? Do you think you're better than we are?"

Such social pressure from friends or family members can be deadly in its power, bolstering every thought you ever had that your problem is intractable and will never go away. How can you break free of dysfunctional eating patterns if there's a chance that by doing so you might hurt others' feelings or risk losing their love?

The Permitter is very important, then, for he or she ritualistically permits you to break free of the chains that bind you. This person can say with genuine sincerity that he or she wishes you well as you make the journey to conscious weight loss, and is happy that you have found your way to this point. He or she absolves you of any and every feeling of guilt that you might be leaving anyone behind as you take this step. Rather, this individual congratulates and thanks you for providing an example of liberation to those who are ready to be liberated, too.

The request to both your Inspirer and your Permitter should be made with seriousness of intent, as this step is no insignificant matter. You will make it clear that nothing is demanded of them other than (1) presence and participation in your initiation ceremony, and (2) continued goodwill. Yet the request should be made to people whom you know in your heart will join you in this effort with a serious and sincere frame of mind.

If you can't come up with any possible members of your initiation team right now, that's fine. Just allow the desire to find them to stay alive in your heart. The time will come, either a minute from now or weeks from now, when the realization of who would be perfect for both jobs will blaze forth within your mind. When you are ready, their names will emerge. You will not rush to ask them, perhaps, but will allow the spirit within you to guide the process. There is no rush to any of this; rather, you're learning to attune yourself to a more natural flow of things.

It's no accident that such attunement will ultimately apply to a more natural flow of eating. From who should be on your team, to what book might appear in your life to help you take a next step, to food that would be a gift to you rather than a source of suffering, the universe supports you in your path toward health and healing. This isn't because you're special, or because overeating is somehow different from other forms of wounding. It is because the universe itself is an expression of Divine love.

The universe is a perfect work of infinite genius, ever creative, life sustaining, and restorative. And its principle of perfection is built into everything. As you realign your mind with Spirit, every cell of your being will return to its natural perfection; in time it will guide you toward every right answer, every right choice, and every right morsel of food.

You are now beginning a new chapter in the cultivation of your highest expression as a human being. You are embarking upon a journey to your higher self, a journey that will both set you free and keep you free.

Let us now ritualize the change in you.

With both your Inspirer and your Permitter beside you, go to your altar and remove the piece of fruit you placed there in Lesson 6. (For purposes of this exercise, we're going to say that it is an apple.) Place the fruit on a plate in front of you.

Your ceremony now involves three things: a statement from you, a statement from your Inspirer, and a statement from your Permitter.

Each person is free to write and say what is in his or her own heart, but here are some statements that evoke the power of the initiation ritual:

You

With this ceremony, I hereby state that I am ready to embark on a new journey in my life. I do not do this without trepidation. I freely admit my fear, but I embrace my faith as well. I am calling on a power within me that can do for me what I cannot do for myself, to help me leave behind a terrible compulsion and lead me to a new way of life.

How I think about food . . . how I think about my body . . . how I eat . . . how I treat my body . . . these subjects have become overwhelming for me, but I surrender them to God. I request a miracle. I pray for freedom, and I thank my friends for being here with me, praying as I pray and holding the vision of my release into a new and better life.

Amen.

Your Inspirer

Dear [your name],

I am honored to stand here today, as a symbol of all those who wish for you a total healing. As one who is free when it comes to food, I pray that my freedom be shared with you. I wish for you a happy, healthy relationship with food and a happy, healthy relationship with your body.

I speak to you as from the other side of a river that you now stand before, both beckoning you and inviting you to cross to a new land within yourself.

I embrace God's promise that you shall be released, and I envision you in sweet and holy freedom. I hold that vision within my heart; I will hold it always and I shall not waver.

May you be blessed on your journey, and may my blessing remain with you as a light upon your path.

Your Permitter

Dear [your name],

Congratulations on the step you are taking today. I wish you well. While I myself have not yet embarked upon (or completed) my journey to conscious weight loss, I am genuinely happy that you are making yours. I know that your success increases my own chances, and

I surrender—on behalf of anyone who might feel this way—any jealousy or other negative feelings projected onto you as you make your break for freedom.

As you leave behind the pain of compulsive eating, know that I—and many others, too—wish you well in your efforts. On behalf of all of us, I wish you love and peace as you make this journey. Most important, I pray for your success. I pray for your recovery and release. I pray that you receive a miracle.

After the third person has spoken, take a knife—a nice one, by the way; no plastic!—and cut your apple into three pieces. Give one piece to your Inspirer, one to your Permitter, and keep one for yourself. Now all three of you are to eat a piece of the apple, symbolizing the role that each of you plays in an effort that will now bear fruit.

Reflection and Prayer

Today's reflection is a continuation of your initiation ceremony. Spend two or three minutes in silence with your Inspirer and Permitter, as well as anyone else you have asked to witness the ceremony. Allow everyone present to offer their words of support.

Close your ceremony with a prayer.

Dear God,
As I enter into this new chapter
of my life,
please bless my steps forward.
With this ceremony,
may Your Spirit come upon me
and release me from my former self.
Please deliver me to sweeter realms
and teach me how to be, dear God,
a freer person, a happier person,
a saner person,
without compulsion or fear.
And so it is.
Amen

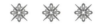

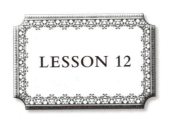

COMMIT
TO YOURSELF

Every overeater has heard them a million times: the admonishments of weight loss. You've got to stick to your diet, commit to the process, stay with it no matter what, discipline yourself to "just do it," and so forth. Yet such admonishments only add to your anxiety; if you were able to consistently *be there* for yourself, you wouldn't be an overeater to begin with!

While overeating would be seen by some as an indulgence of self, it is in fact a profound *rejection* of self. It is a moment of self-betrayal and self-punishment, and anything *but* a commitment to one's own well-being. Why would you be able to commit to a diet if you're not already consistently committed to yourself?

Your relationship to food is a reflection of your relationship to yourself, as is everything in your life. There's no reason to think that you'll be capable of loyalty to a diet until you address your basic disloyalty toward yourself. Until your fundamental relationship with yourself is healed, then your relationship to food is doomed to be neurotic.

As committed as you might be to the process of weight loss, there will always come those moments when your self-hatred rises up like an oceanic force from the bottom of your subconscious mind, demanding to assert itself. That's what makes addiction and compulsion so cruel: you could be committed to your diet for 23 hours and 45 minutes during a day, then ruin all your efforts in 15 minutes.

What is not self-love carries within it the seeds of self-hate, no matter how small; wherever the mind is not filled with love, it has a propensity for insanity. And just a tiny bit of insanity is enough to do it—in about as long as it takes to open up a bag of cookies, you find a way to destroy your most cherished dream.

This lesson addresses your basic lack of commitment and compassion toward yourself, your lack of self-care that leads you time and again to punish and betray yourself. Only when you learn to commit to yourself will you stop your self-sabotaging behavior. It's not enough to just tell yourself what not to do; you must learn a new way to *think* before you can master a new way to *be*. In the last lesson, you asked others to stand up for you; with this lesson, you will learn to stand up for yourself.

All of us wish we'd had perfect childhoods, with a mother and father who modeled ideal parental attitudes and taught us to internalize the tenets of self-love. Many of us, however, did not. Perhaps you grew up with no one to model for you that you were truly valuable, that your thoughts were appreciated, that your feelings deserved tending to, or that your worth was deeply appreciated. And whatever *was* modeled—positive or negative—became the model for your relationship with your adult self. That is simply how adult personas form.

If you were neglected as a child, you learned to neglect yourself as an adult. If you were betrayed as a child, you learned to betray yourself as an adult. If no one cared about your feelings as a child, you didn't know how to care for your own feelings once you became an adult. Maybe on some level your parents weren't *there* for you; and now, in the moment when you overeat, you simply repeat the pattern by failing to be there for yourself.

Or your parent or parents might have loved you very much yet simply lacked the psychological tools to help you build an emotionally healthy relationship with yourself. It's only recently, in historical terms, that society has even considered the possibility that children have valuable thoughts of their own. Looking back into your childhood isn't about figuring out whom you can blame, or building a case to justify feelings of victimization. It's simply about identifying your wound so the medicine of love can be applied correctly.

A way to repair a broken childhood is to allow God to re-parent you. As a child, you had no choice but to depend on your parents' love . . . and where it was twisted or absent, you suffered accordingly. Yet now you are no longer a child, and can redo your childhood by remembering Whose child you truly are.

By seeing that you are a child of God—by recognizing the unwavering love and mercy He extends to you every moment of the day—you begin to realign your attitudes toward yourself with His attitudes toward you. You no longer need to model anyone's neglect of you; you need only model God's love for you.

As you reestablish the Divine connection that was severed by any wounding in your childhood, your mind begins to move away from thoughts that weaken you and instead think thoughts that strengthen you. You will learn to *be there* for yourself, and in a moment when you are there for yourself, you simply don't *want* to behave self-destructively. It won't be so hard to commit to right eating once you've recommitted to yourself. It will be natural. Appetites that reflect an unloving attitude toward yourself will simply fall by the wayside, like leaves in autumn when their season is done.

This is a *re*commitment in that you were born with your connection to your true self intact; while this connection might have been broken in your experience, it was never broken in the mind of God. In Alcoholics Anonymous, there is reference to "conscious contact." Your contact with the Divine is still there; it is simply no longer conscious. And by bringing it back into full awareness, you will reconnect with it experientially. Like a plug that has dropped to the floor, your mind needs to be plugged back into the socket that provides its true sense of self.

Grounded in our Divine nature, every human being tends naturally toward connection, creativity, and joy. Such is the natural flow of the human experience, just as the bud flows naturally into the fullness of a rose blossom. The difference between you and the rose is that, as a human being, you have a *choice* as to whether or not to let your blossoming occur. If the rosebud were somehow able to deny the blossom the right to emerge, then what would happen to the energy that would have turned it into a blossom? Is it *un*created? Does it go away? No, because energy cannot be uncreated.

When a natural flow of energy is denied, it turns into a kind of backward flow, or implosion of identity. You are then tempted to misdirect your creative passion.

If you deny yourself your own passion, your own path, your own longing, your own drama, your own life force, your own truth—then you might be tempted to live vicariously through those who allow themselves theirs. Your creative energy has got to go *somewhere*, even if it is projected onto others. You're tempted to live a life of fantasy if you deny yourself a life of truth.

It's an easy path from a whole box of chocolates to immersion in the latest tabloid, from denying yourself your own drama to drinking in the drama of others. But it's not as though others were programmed for exciting lives and you weren't. For whatever reason, some people were simply not blocked in childhood the way that you were. They can more easily allow themselves to experience the natural, creative drama of their own lives.

Think of the person whose life you look at and secretly think, *Oh, I wish that were my life.* Now imagine yourself in kindergarten with that individual. Use your inner eye to face the truth here, and you will see that at the age of five, he or she had nothing on you. You came into this life with the same creative energy and the same Divine programming that everyone else has. And you still have it; it's simply backed up, taking anti-expression in the form of excess flesh.

But all that can be corrected now. A valve that has been closed can now be reopened. A habit—and that is all it is: a bad mental habit—can be unlearned and replaced by your natural, spiritual proclivity to go forth into the world and create the good, the true, and the beautiful.

You should be committed to yourself because God is committed to you. How else but through the thoughts that naturally emerge within you can He impress Himself upon your soul? In listening to yourself, you're tuning in to the vibrations of Spirit that are the natural communication of the Creator with the created.

God doesn't have a plan for Miss America, but not for you. God doesn't have a plan for some movie star, but not for you. There is a Divine plan by which each and every person's life is programmed for the highest level of creativity and goodness and truth. There are roses and daisies and peonies and violets, all very different but all very beauti-ful. Nature sees each of us as expressions of itself, and to accept that expression, to honor the natural flow of your own thoughts and feelings, is not just a gift you give your-self—it is your gift to the world.

Try to forgive those who in their ignorance sought to block your truth, whether five minutes ago or 40 years ago. And try to forgive yourself for all the years you have failed to listen to yourself.

When you grasp excessively for anything in this world—and for you that happens to be food—you deny what is try-ing to emerge from deep within you. Failing to experience what is *supposed* to happen—your own internal communion with self—you are thrown into an awful, primordial void, bereft by what feels like the absence of your Creator. You don't really mean to be grasping for food. You mean to be grasping for God. And there is only one way to do that. You cannot find Him except where He lives. And He lives in you.

For this lesson you will use your journal pages, begin-ning a process by which you'll learn to support yourself . . . befriend yourself . . . commit to yourself. You'll start by learning to dialogue with yourself, asking and receiving the truth of what you think and how you feel.

With every journal entry, you'll have a conversation with yourself that is long overdue:

1. You to self: *What are your thoughts?*

This question shows that you care what your own thoughts are. You value them.

If, when you were a child, no one seemed to care what you thought, then you developed a habit of not listening to yourself any more than those around you did. Perhaps you were teased for your beliefs by a parent or sibling, teaching you to deem your own thoughts valueless. If either of those situations occurred, it would have severed your connection to self in a most fundamental way. If you don't listen to yourself, you can't honor yourself. If you don't listen to yourself, you can't hear God's voice within you. If you don't listen to yourself, you program your body to stop listening to *itself*. And thus the hell that follows.

In your journal pages, morning and evening, write down your thoughts of the day. Your writing will become a conscious repository for thoughts you would have formerly discounted. You speak, and someone listens.

Whatever thoughts you can remember—whether you consider them significant or routine—write them down and allow yourself to see, review, and bear witness to them all. They aren't good or bad; they just *are*. What is important is that they are yours. Any positive thought obviously needs to be heard by you. And any negative thought needs to be heard by you as well, to be learned from perhaps and then surrendered for healing. Both thoughts and feelings matter, and we will discuss feelings more thoroughly in the next lesson.

What matters now is that you realize that it's right, not wrong, to listen to yourself. In the moment you overeat, it's not just that an inappropriate dynamic is present; it's that a healthy dynamic is absent. By learning to build anew the dynamics of a healthy self-regard, the craziness of your compulsion is cut off at the pass.

2. You to self: *I forgive you for your mistakes.*

In the words of the famed Jewish sage Hillel the Elder: "If I am not for myself, then who will be for me? And if I am only for myself, then what am I?"

This lesson speaks to the first of those questions—your need to show compassion for yourself as a prerequisite for attracting compassion from others. If you are angry at yourself, then your body will register that negativity. Your body, remember, is a reflection of your thoughts. As long as you withhold love from yourself, your body will appear to withhold love from you.

If you didn't receive much mercy as a child—if mistakes were met with a lack of forgiveness or you were repeatedly told you weren't worthy or good—then overeating is a reenactment of the message, "You're bad! You're bad!" The fork or spoon with which you overeat is not something with which you gift yourself, but rather a whip with which you punish yourself. And once you realize what you've done, once you see that you've fallen off the wagon again, then you're thrown into a new cycle of anger—anger at yourself for overeating!

In your journal pages, morning and evening, write down whatever you feel were mistakes, but then surrender them. Explore the feelings of both remorse and self-forgiveness. Feel the pain of knowing you've made a mistake, but also the extraordinary relief that comes over your spirit once you've atoned for your error and surrendered it to an all-merciful God.

When you overeat, you show a lack of mercy for yourself. By reclaiming the compassion that is natural to your true self, you will learn to eat moderately as an expression of self-love. If and when you fall off the wagon—times when, despite your efforts, you can't resist the urge to eat self-destructively—you will begin to say "Oops" with a lighthearted acceptance rather than a groan of despair. And that will decrease the chances that it will happen again, for you will have stopped fueling self-hate with more self-hate.

3. You to self: *I think your dreams are important.*

A healthy person is constantly dreaming up the next best thing . . . from what video would be fun to watch tonight, to whom it would be good to call on the telephone later, to where it would be pleasurable to go for the weekend. But if you don't listen to yourself, then how do you *know* what you think is the right place to go or the right thing to do? And if you don't know the right thing, then you're prone to doing the wrong thing. And that includes what you eat and don't eat.

Someone somewhere didn't listen to your heart, and as a consequence you stopped listening to it, too. Not in every area of life, perhaps; in many areas you might be very functional, even supremely successful. But your subconscious mind chose an available tool by which to express the deeper truth of a hidden self-hatred.

The voice of the discounting or belittling grown-up has remained, for it has not yet been ushered out. As a consequence, you subconsciously follow the dictates of a ghost. You still punish yourself; you still deny yourself; you still discount yourself. And so it goes. The idea that you can fight such a force by simply sticking to a diet is almost silly.

In your journal pages, morning and evening, dialogue with yourself about your true dreams. From going to Paris to looking beautiful, from writing a book to owning your own business, from having a mate to having children, what do you really long for? What do you really wish to be true for you? What is your heart's desire . . . for if *you* won't honor it, then who else will?

It doesn't matter that Mommy or Daddy or your siblings or your teachers or whoever else didn't value your dreams. God did, and He does. It's time for you to start thinking like God whenever you think about anything . . . including yourself.

This journaling process is an important tool, and not just for losing weight. It's a tool for cultivating your highest *self,* as applied not only to weight but to any area of your life. Journaling is a way you listen to yourself, by making it clear to yourself what you actually think and feel. The more space you give yourself to express your real thoughts and feelings, the more your wisdom will emerge. In listening to yourself, you *learn* from yourself. In listening deeply to the voice of your heart, you reestablish relationship with your true self, so long denied.

Start listening to yourself now and you will find that what you hear is the music of your soul. Its sounds will accompany you as you move toward the life, and the body, that nature intends for you. In the eyes of God, you are more beautiful than you realize and more cherished than you know.

Reflection and Prayer

The reflection that accompanies this lesson is a flow of consciousness to apply to every moment of your life. Instead of asking yourself, "What do you think?" and providing the answer only twice a day during a journaling session, begin to dialogue naturally with yourself throughout the day.

Remind yourself in every moment how important it is for you to be in touch with your own thoughts and feelings. From that place only, will you honor deeply enough the thoughts and feelings of others. If you deny yourself, you will always deny other people. But by connecting to your own truth, you will begin to connect more deeply with the truth in others. Through that connection, you will free yourself from a false connection to food. At that point, food will be become as important as it is meant to be—no more and no less.

Dear God,
Please show me how to honor myself.
Please teach me how to listen to myself.
Please program my mind to know itself,
that I might at last be free.
Teach me to appreciate
Your Spirit that lives within me.
Show me how to be good to myself,
that I might know more fully
the goodness of life.
Amen

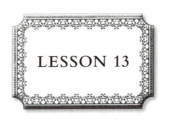

FEEL YOUR FEELINGS

We've already established that the subconscious force of food compulsion is made up of unprocessed feelings. You seek, when you overeat, to contain the emotions that swirl within you—to put them somewhere, to put a lid on them, or to make yourself numb so you won't have to feel them at all.

What makes your emotions different, remember, is not *what* you feel. What makes your emotions different is how you process them . . . and sometimes how you *cannot* process them. For the food addict, feelings that can and should be processed in the mind are often displaced onto the body, where they cannot be processed and therefore remain stored within your flesh.

The only way to remove the weight of unprocessed feelings is to allow yourself to actually feel them. Once again, childhood patterns are the issue. Someone else's love and understanding—and for a child, that someone else is the parent—provides a container for our feelings. Later in life, if such a container were absent in childhood, the overeater tends to seek through excessive eating the containment that food cannot give.

Parental love is meant to be a model for Divine love. When parental love holds us safe, we more easily transfer as adults to a sense that we are safe in the arms of the Divine. If you didn't feel that you could safely take your feelings to your parent figure, it's doubtful you feel now that you can give all your feelings to God.

Feelings that are not acknowledged cannot be fully felt. How can you fully feel something that you fail to name? *I feel sad, I feel embarrassed, I feel overwhelmed, I feel humiliated, I feel angry, I feel afraid, I feel rejected, I feel left out, I feel betrayed, I feel wronged, I feel insulted, I feel hopeless, I feel anxious, I feel frustrated, I feel guilty, I feel lonely* . . . too often translate into: *I feel hungry.*

Darn right you're hungry, but not for food. Having bypassed even a conscious recognition of your pain, you went straight for a way to assuage it. You're looking to an external source to provide an experience that can only be found internally. You can't get rid of your pain without admitting to yourself that it's there.

Emotions need to be *felt* the way that food needs to be chewed; emotions need to be digested within your psyche the way food is digested in your stomach. The compulsive eater often gorges on food as a way to avoid feeling feelings, but then treats food the same way he or she treated the emotion—moving too quickly, failing to chew, and failing to properly digest it.

Once your feelings are felt, they can be acknowledged, looked at, learned from, and surrendered to Divine Mind. But instead of acknowledging and *feeling* your feelings, you've learned to discount them before they can even rise up fully formed. You suppress what you're too afraid to feel, having little or no trust in the wisdom of your emotions.

You don't know your emotions *have* any wisdom—how could you, given that no one honored them when you were a child? But they do; they are part of the genius of the human psyche.

Emotions, even painful ones, are here to tell you something. They are messages to be tended to. Yet how can you tend to something you don't know is there? Emotions must be acknowledged and *felt;* or else they cannot be learned from, grown from, or processed.

Life might have taught you that emotions are dangerous. Perhaps as a child, you were told things such as, "Don't you cry or I'll give you something to cry about!"—an emotionally tyrannical message that certainly would have taught you to suppress your feelings at all costs. Perhaps your emotions were ignored, minimized, or even laughed at by parents who had other things and other children to think about. What matters is that, for whatever reason, you learned at a very young age to neither honor nor even really feel your own feelings.

In an earlier lesson, we explored the effects of trauma. If you experienced severe, even violent, trauma, you learned to automatically numb yourself so as not to feel the next blow. It was a brilliant coping mechanism on the part of your subconscious mind, to freeze so quickly that when the blow came, you would already be numb.

The problem, however, is that such a coping mechanism was only intended for emergency purposes; it was manufactured to save you from imminent danger, not to take you through life. It was not meant to fundamentally alter your system of emotional responses, and yet that is what occurred.

At a very young age you were exposed to what your psyche perceived as danger, and now your subconscious mind does not make a distinction between dangerous threat and tolerable stress. It doesn't know what to let in and what to guard against, so it guards against *everything,* just in case.

Central to the holistic healing of your weight issue is that you develop a new skill set with which to deal with unpleasant emotions. An emotion swept under the rug is not an emotion that goes away; it's simply an emotion that is put somewhere other than where it should be put. It becomes inert rather than dynamic energy, stored within you rather than being released.

As noted previously, energy cannot be uncreated. And emotions are powerful forms of energy. If you're too frightened to feel a feeling, its energy still has to go somewhere. Actually, an emotion is not dangerous *until* it's disowned, for that's when it commonly gets projected onto others and/or compressed into your own flesh. That only produces more feelings—shame, humiliation, embarrassment, and failure—resulting in an endless barrage of twisted reasons telling you why you might as well just give up and eat more.

Defending against being overwhelmed by your emotions, you actually create emotions that are overwhelming. You begin by trying to keep your emotions at bay, eat them, go numb instead of feeling them—and in so doing, create a situation that causes you an endless run of painful emotions. By trying to escape your feelings, you create a whole slew of them that will arrive full force once you realize what you've done. The only feelings you really need to fear are those you ignore.

In Greek mythology, Poseidon is god of the sea. If he tells the waves to calm down, then the waves calm down. In the New Testament, Jesus walked onto the water and stopped the storm. Both are metaphysical descriptions of the effects of Divine Mind on the storms of the inner self. Spirit is the master, not the slave, of the inner sea. Your task, therefore, is to give your feelings to God, that you might be lifted above the storms of your subconscious mind. The storms are raging for one reason only: your inner self will not be ignored.

Your thinking that you alone can control the overwhelming force of unprocessed feelings is like a small child thinking he or she can stand on the beach and make the waves stop. You might grit your teeth and make it through the morning; you might white-knuckle it and make it through lunchtime; you might even somehow be able to make it till 10 P.M. But at some point, the now angry wave of "I will be fed"—"How *dare* you say 'No' to me? How *dare* you say 'No'?!"—will catch you by the ankles and drag you to the kitchen or whatever place you keep your stash. And the craving, once more, will win.

Your craving for food is an emotional temper tantrum, as a part of you that feels unheard is demanding to be heard and *will* be heard. You have two choices: you can feel your emotion, or you can listen to the cruel command to do something to temporarily assuage the pain of not feeling it. Clearly, feeling the emotion would be a more functional choice.

If you have no template for honoring feelings, processing them, bearing witness to them, surrendering them, and watching them miraculously transform, then they can appear in your life as frightening energy ruling you instead of being ruled by you. It's time to end your emotional slavery by building your spiritual mastery.

Spiritual mastery does not emerge from self-will but from surrender of self-will. Once you've felt a feeling and surrendered it, you are not simply left with it, as if you're dangling from an emotional cliff and about to fall into an abyss from which you can never escape. When you give a painful emotion to Divine Mind, you give it to a power that can take it from you by changing the thoughts that produced it.

Anything you surrender for Divine transformation will be transformed, and anything you cling to will not be transformed. Surrendering your feelings involves feeling them first, yes, but then it involves giving them up.

It's actually ironic that you should be afraid of feeling your feelings; as an overeater, what you have created for yourself and have had to endure are some of the most painful emotions there are. The horrible feelings of failure that are endemic to the chronic overeater make your tolerance for pain already higher than you think. The pain you're trying to avoid is nothing compared to the pain you've already lived through.

The Swiss psychologist Carl Jung said: "All neurosis is a substitute for legitimate suffering." Any pathological tendency—overeating included—represents the twisted energies of unprocessed pain. The pathology is not ended by suppressing your pain, but by feeling the legitimate suffering it is seeking to express.

Spiritual healing is a process. First you feel the feeling; then you feel whatever pain might legitimately arise from it; then you pray to learn whatever lesson the pain can teach you; then you seek to forgive; and, at last, the grace of God is given you. You emerge from the experience no longer suffering, and having grown as a human being. When you are more attuned to growing spiritually, you need not grow so much physically. The energy is released and let out, no longer pushed into your flesh.

You're afraid of feelings the way you're afraid of food: you're afraid that once you start, you may never stop. But the truth is, feelings are only out of control when they're *not* handed over for Divine resolution. Given to Divine Mind, they're lifted to Divine right order—where they will be appropriately felt and then appropriately dissolved. So too shall it be with food appetites, for they are mere reflections of your turmoil or peace.

The fact that a feeling is painful is not necessarily a reason to avoid it. Perhaps you did something to sabotage yourself in a relationship; unless you feel the remorse, how will you recognize your self-destructive pattern? Perhaps your husband left you; your sadness is understandable given that you were married for 30 years. Perhaps your child is seriously ill; your grief and fear are simply signs that you are human.

These feelings, when handled appropriately, become stations on the way to grace. Yes, you will emerge as someone who has grown and will no longer self-sabotage, but *first you had to feel the pain.* Yes, you will emerge from your divorce strong and free to love again, but *first you had to feel the pain.* Yes, you will become the warrior parent who takes charge of your child's healing, but *first you had to feel the pain.*

Your suffering does not make you weak; only your avoidance of suffering makes you weak. And that avoidance—the avoidance of legitimate suffering—is unfortunately bolstered by the cultural attitudes of a society obsessed with cheap and easy happiness.

Several years ago, one of my daughter's teenage friends— a golden boy of extraordinary beauty, talent, intelligence, and kindness—shot and killed himself with his father's hunting rifle. There were so many aspects of the situation rife with horror (including his having been one more statistic involving the connection between teenage use of antidepressants and suicide). As a mother, I felt, as did all the parents in my daughter's circle of friends, a deep concern for my child's pain.

I remember telling my shattered, darling girl, her face streaming with tears, that there are some times in life when the worst thing that could possibly happen does happen. I told her that Robbie's death was a full-tilt catastrophe, and nothing I could say would change that. That Robbie was alive forever in the arms of God, but that didn't make this human tragedy any less horrible. That every tear she felt like crying was a tear she had to cry, and she would know when she had cried enough when she didn't have any more tears left.

I remember seeing a look of relief on my daughter's face when I told her this; she needed desperately to be given permission to feel her feelings and not suppress them. Indeed, I cried with her. The last thing I ever would have wanted to do is delegitimize or circumvent her grief.

I remember saying at a grief support group I led years ago for people who had lost their loved ones, "Hey, guys, remember. This is a grief *support* group, not a grief *denial* group." Grief is a way that our emotional ecosystem, imbued with the same genius as every other aspect of nature, processes an otherwise too shocking emotional reality.

The fact that you are sad doesn't inherently mean that something's wrong. It simply means that you are sad. It simply means that you are human. Regardless of what your feeling is, it simply *is*.

There is no reason to run to food—or to anything else, for that matter—to escape your feelings. Your feelings are not your enemy but your friend. They always have something to teach you—even the tough ones. Sadness handled gracefully will transform into peace, but only if you allow yourself to feel it first. That is the core message of every great religious and spiritual system in the world: that the story isn't over until the happy part.

My daughter would get to the point of peaceful acceptance of Robbie's death, and even a spiritual realization at the idea that one day she would see him again. But none of that could have come about in a real and authentic way had she not first allowed herself to feel the incredible grief of his untimely death.

164

Another feeling the overeater commonly seeks to avoid is the simple stress of living in the modern world. From running a household to running a company, the stress of our modern existence has people running for whatever form of anesthetization they can find. *I eat because I feel overwhelmed.* The feeling of overwhelm is a natural consequence of failing to recognize a Divine hand holding all things together.

If you feel you must control everything by yourself—if you don't feel you can ask for God's help with the details—then no wonder you feel absolutely overwhelmed. You can't exactly hold up the stars in the sky, but obviously *someone* does. So couldn't that someone hold and harmonize the circumstances of your life?

In fact, the entire universe is held safely in Divine hands. Planets revolve around the sun, stars stay in the sky, cells divide, and embryos turn into babies. Embryos don't exclaim, "I don't know how I'm going to do this! I don't know how to cell-divide!" The embryo doesn't *have* to know. An order bigger than the embryo moves it forward as part of nature's blueprint.

Any situation placed in Divine hands is lifted to Divine right order. If looking at the stars in a starry sky doesn't overwhelm you, then neither should your own circumstances. They are put together, held together, and corrected when need be by the same loving force.

But *unless* you feel how overwhelmed you are—unless you can say, "Wow, I'm feeling overwhelmed right now . . . I feel like this whole thing could fall apart if I even closed my eyes for a second"—then you're not in a position to surrender it. Pray for the following miracle:

Dear God,
Please take this situation.
I place it in Your hands.
Please handle all the details,
heal my mind of error,
and reveal to me what You would have me do.
Amen

You need not carry the weight of the world either on your spirit *or* on your body. You can "lighten up," because the spirit is with you. Give over your burdens, and journey lightly through the world.

Every emotion, every situation, every relationship, and every issue can be safely given to Divine Mind for upliftment. The purpose of this lesson is to move your mind from its habit of suppressing your emotions—whatever they are—to the comfort and peace of surrendering them to God.

Reflection and Prayer

For this lesson, you need a God Box.

It might be a box you make, a box you buy, or a box you previously used for some other purpose. But as with other tools used in this course, this box should be beautiful. It is something that will be put on the altar and given to God. It is a container within which a miraculous process will occur.

Now take a piece of paper and write down these sentences:

"Give Me your pain, and I will take it from you."

— GOD

"Place all of this in My hands."

— GOD

"Seek to forgive, and you will have peace."

— G O D

*"You are My perfect creation. Nothing you
have ever done or thought, and nothing anyone
else has done or thought, changes that fact."*

— G O D

"Give Me your errors, and I will correct them for you."

— G O D

*"You are deeply loved. Nothing you
do can change My love for you."*

— G O D

Add to these sentences any scriptural or inspirational quotes that appeal to you, including any ideas of your own, and put them in your God Box.

Your job is to continually review your emotions, admit them, feel them, write them down, and give them to Divine Mind. Use your journal pages to specifically describe and explore an emotion, and then simply write: "Dear God, I surrender this feeling to You." Then go to your altar, and for every emotion you surrender, open your God Box and blindly pick out a saying. It will tell you what you need to hear.

Now you're ready to meditate. You have surrendered your feelings, and your mind will now be imbued with wisdom. This will bring you peace.

Honoring your feelings on a regular basis, you will build the attitudinal strength to carry you when an emotional storm arises in your subconscious sea. Before you walk into the kitchen, you will name your emotion, even if you have to scream it. Before you drive to the hamburger stand, you will say, "God, please help me," even if at that moment you don't believe there is a God. Before you drown in the deep and toxic waters of your craving, you will feel your feelings and surrender them to God, even if you do so with but a mustard seed of faith.

Your God Box will help you. It will provide answers. And in time, you will heal.

Dear God,
I give to You my anguish and my sorrow.
I feel so overwhelmed, dear God,
by my life and my compulsion.
Take from me my craving, dear God,
for I cannot fight it and I feel so weak.
Show me how to feel my feelings
and to surrender them to You.
Restore my spirit
and give me strength.
Thank You, God.
Amen

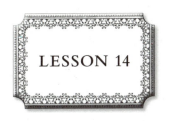

ALLOW THE PAIN

This lesson refers to the emotional detoxification process that accompanies serious weight loss. At a certain point in your journey, feelings that have been denied, repressed, and/or impacted within you begin rising up in order to be released.

In the last lesson, we discussed how feelings are not good or bad; they simply are. But that doesn't mean they're not painful. It's one thing to know that suffering is an inevitable part of the human journey, but it's another thing altogether to learn how to cope with it.

With any spiritual journey—and the journey to conscious weight loss *is* a spiritual journey—things often seem to get worse before they get better. Love's light is being shined on many places heretofore not visible to your conscious mind, revealing toxic feelings that were there already but cleverly hidden.

It's all right if this part of your journey is not pleasant. Part of your repatterning is learning to be with unpleasantness in a healthy way. The mature and sober person knows that on some days things simply feel rotten, and *that is okay*. You are learning to move through distress by simply being with it, without the need to overeat or to act out in any other way.

How could it not be unpleasant, having to refeel feelings that you've been eating for years? Now having to confront them, deal with them, and ultimately accept them feels like a fever within your soul.

But a spiritual fever, like a physical fever, actually has a productive function: it burns up disease. Think of your pain as a feverish burning up of fear. As you heal physically, extreme fever can lead to delirium. And as you heal spiritually, your fever can lead to delirium as well—a quiet delirium of the soul. But this too shall pass.

This lesson concerns itself with human despair and the consistency of the body's cells. Man has looked beneath the surface of the skin for centuries, probing the internal workings of the human body. During the last century, science has developed the ability to view even the tiniest cells that make up our physical tissue. Yet science has not yet discovered an explanation for how emotional change produces physical change, and it is particularly blind to the malleability of fat.

In fact, there are many levels of understanding—even of our physical selves—that science has not yet penetrated. An electron microscope reveals the entire picture of our cellular system, but within the cells themselves, there are storehouses of information not yet understood.

For instance, there are tears and then there are tears. Some varieties are toxic to the body, while others are healing. The distinction between the two is not just an emotional difference but a physical one as well. Even materially, there are aspects to tears—including functions that affect the workings of the brain—that have not yet been scientifically identified.

Sometimes it's only through crying tears that need to be shed that we dissolve the unhappiness that caused them. That is why *suppressing* unhappiness doesn't tend to end it. How many times have we said that someone "needs a good cry." Indeed. Toxicity is often released through the tear ducts as part of the body's natural genius at flushing itself out. Casual use of antidepressants is unwise for just this reason— feeling the full extent of your sadness is sometimes the only way to heal it. In the absence of the feeling, you miss out on the healing. The body does not make distinctions among physical, emotional, psychological, and spiritual stresses. It is equipped with the natural intelligence to address them all.

You are mistaken if you think that you can fundamentally and permanently change bodily symptoms by physical means alone. *Problems must leave through the same door they came in.* If mistaken thoughts have created a problem, then righting those thoughts is essential to healing it. And if toxic feelings created a problem, they can only leave through a detox process by which they come up again in order to be released.

Fat is not just inert cellular tissue. It is a repository of twisted, distorted thoughts and feelings that didn't have anywhere else to go. If you remove the fat tissue but do not remove its psychic cause, then the fat might go but the causal imprint remains. And the imprint, in time, will attract more substance with which to materially express itself.

It's not enough to just "lose your weight." You must lose the emotional weight that lurks behind it. This you have already begun to do. Remember that your food compulsion is a way to cope with painful feelings. As you begin to heal from those feelings—removing their "imprint" from your consciousness—they are necessarily *refelt* on their way out.

Problems that seem to have nothing to do with your weight issues might rise up, and in particularly challenging forms. You might doubt yourself in ways you have not done before, or have not done for a very long time. But this part of your process is not a bad period; it is actually a good one, for it is necessary. There is no spiritual rehabilitation without this kind of detoxification.

When any pain, difficulty, frustration, or challenge emerges, try to see it, honor it, bear witness to it, and receive it as part of your healing. The situation carries within it important information for you. It is not just randomly happening at this time. It presents the opportunity to examine critically important issues in your life. Looking at your pain, feeling the feelings, learning whatever lessons are being brought up for review—these are ultimately the only ways to get the pain to burn away.

The universe will never leave you alone at such a time as this. Angels are all around you, as they gather without fail whenever a soul is seeking its wholeness. This is absolutely not the time to isolate; rather, despite whatever resistance you feel, allow yourself to join with at least one other human being who might possibly be able to help you. You will learn the serious value of sacred friendship and/or professional counseling.

Perhaps you will attend support groups, or spontaneously create a small community of like-minded souls all taking this journey together. Books might fall off the shelf in front of you, and even strangers might have something profound, wise, and relevant to say. Connecting more deeply with others, you will connect more deeply to your own feelings. And even sadness will be more bearable. Some days are sad, yet sad days pass. Spiritual mastery involves building the mental, emotional, and behavioral habits to carry you through such times without an explosion of dysfunctional behavior.

Sometimes you just need to make space for sadness. You do not need an excuse for why you feel sad; you do not need to "fix" it; and, most important, you do not need to run from it. What you need is to let it come up and simply be with it.

Your task with this lesson is to make space in your life, just as you make space in your heart, for any sadness you need to honor. Perhaps take a walk each evening, or a stroll on the beach each morning. Allow yourself to grieve.

You will learn in time to *be* with the void, addressing it with a bubble bath rather than a sandwich, and with prayer time rather than a candy bar. Your task is to inhabit the emptiness, breathe through it, learn its lessons, and hear the message it conveys. There is no hole for you to try to fill with food or anything else; there is only the primal void within every human being when we feel we cannot find God.

Great literature, particularly tales of true tragedy, can be cathartic; it gives a voice to your own buried, free-floating sadness, and provides a conduit for its dissolution. When you read *Anna Karenina* in college, really, what did you know? But now, after you've known a few Vronskys of your own, you read the book with a new understanding: your pain is given meaning there, immortalized in a character living precisely your own heartbreak. And in Anna's response to her despair, you get to see the stark reality that confronts you now: you can self-destruct, or you can rise up in glory.

You did not become an overeater for no reason. If you choose to honestly confront the emotions involved in both causing and healing your compulsive patterns, you *will* experience a dark night of the soul. But a dark night of the soul is ultimately a good thing, for it both precedes and prepares your spirit for rebirth. The darkness is simply the revisiting of old feelings, in the absence of which true healing cannot occur. It's important to remember that this darkness is temporary, and leads ultimately to the light beyond it.

This time must simply be endured. But it is also to be honored for the opportunity it gives you to burn through feelings that have come up at last, and only now can truly leave. They are not being suppressed this time; they are being led to the door. They have been embedded in your flesh, and will now be cast out of your personal universe. The tears you cry now will lead ultimately to rejoicing, as the day will come when you feel the lightness—both physically and spiritually—of a brand-new day.

There are poems, films, and novels—and nonfiction books as well—that give meaning to the experience of deep sorrow. Choose three that speak to you; perhaps something you've already experienced, or a book or movie that you know about but have not yet read or viewed. Place them on your altar and commit yourself to reading or viewing them. In honoring them, you honor your own tears in a way that releases rather than suppresses them. Such is the value of art.

Reflection and Prayer

Relax, close your eyes, and pray for comfort.

Give to Divine Mind your despair, your sadness, your hopelessness, your regret, your embarrassment, your pain, your grief, your fear, and your burdens. Do not rush through this darkness. Allow yourself to enter into it in order to move through it. And in time the light will come.

Dear God,
Protect me as I walk through dark hallways of my mind.
Release me from the bondage that would hold me back.
I give to You my hopelessness,
please give to me some hope.
Reveal to me the light of truth,
that my darkness shall disappear.
Each day, send love to guide my heart
and heal my thoughts.
Heal me for Your sake,
and not for mine alone.
Show me how to laugh again
after so long being sad.
Amen

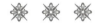

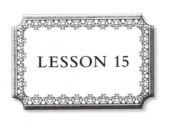

EXIT THE ALONE ZONE

Overeating is not a food issue, but a relationship issue.

Your weight has been, on some level, a statement of your unavailability. Feeling separate from others, you built a wall; then, having built a wall, you felt more separate from others. Separation became a theme, not only regarding your body but in other aspects of your life as well. A wall went up around you physically *and* energetically as you learned to dissociate from others in ways both large and small.

At times you might say an unreasonable "No" to opportunities for human connection; at other times, an overly enthusiastic or needy "Yes" separates you just as much as a "No" would. You've been thrown off track inwardly and outwardly. You must address the issue of your unavailability, or you will not stay on track even if you do get your weight down.

The energetic wall that surrounds you is not visible to the physical eye. It consists of behavioral patterns of which you are probably well aware—and if you aren't, then the people who know you best can surely help identify them.

There is no point in even trying to lose your weight until you have come to the place in your life where you actually *want* to be closer to people. Until that happens, the subconscious urge to build a wall will override any diet you try.

As previously noted, something and/or someone led you to build that wall to begin with. And according to your subconscious mind, you still need protection from that person or event. The subconscious deals in no-time; the fact that the event is long past and the person is long gone represents a rational assessment that means little to the subconscious mind.

Only a miraculous healing, nothing short of the hand of God, is powerful enough to override your primal impulse to protect yourself. That impulse is created by millions of years of evolution; at its core, it represents not dysfunction but the genius of the biological system. The point is that in you, the system was short-circuited and needs to be reset. You are protecting yourself against things that would not hurt you, and failing to protect yourself against things that could.

This lesson focuses on your relationship to other people, as your compulsion is housed in a frozen place you could call your "alone zone." Reaching across whatever wall still divides you from others is essential to your healing, as it helps reverse a dysfunctional pattern by establishing a new one.

A large gun in your fear-mind's arsenal, something that keeps you trapped in the pattern of overeating, is your tendency to isolate. For in isolation you feel permission to self-destruct. There is no one there to say, "Don't do it"; you are free to indulge the deepest craving with no scolding even from yourself, drowned out as a scolding would be by the shrieking and false delights of your compulsion. Once you are alone with the compulsion, you have no power to resist it. And that is why being alone with it is dangerous. You will begin to see that being alone with your compulsion is as dangerous as being alone with a madman, which in a way it is. The compulsion within you *is* madness, and the only antidote to its power is the achievement of deep sanity.

Your problem with weight is calling you to the highest expression of your true self, and your true self is deeply in love with humanity. Each of us carries the tendency to separate ourselves from others. There is such a thing as splendid solitude, but isolation is not it. Isolating is a defense against relationship; and for the overeater, it's the way to avoid dealing with others so that you can have your secret, dark, and sordid relationship with food all by yourself. Food will not pressure you. Food will accept you. Food will understand you. Food will make you feel better. Heroin reads from the same handbook, by the way.

Secret eating holds a goody bag of insanities, from grazing for anything you can find—hot fudge on this cracker might be good!—to standing in front of the fridge and stuffing yourself in the middle of the night. The dark castle of secret eating needs a lock on it, followed by complete demolition.

Author Katherine Woodward Thomas once told me a liberating story about exiting the alone zone. She suffered from food addiction for years when she was young, and at one point found that her toughest problem was night eating.

No matter how much willpower Katherine was able to exert during the day, there was something about the nighttime hours that made her unable to rise above her craving. So she had an idea: she started telling people from her Overeaters Anonymous group that there was a new nighttime-eating hotline, and she gave out its number. Of course the number was hers!

Katherine then spent night after night *helping other people* endure the difficulty of remaining abstinent at night, and in time interrupted the pattern of her own nighttime food hell.

What occurs in such a situation is not an insignificant thing. Reaching out to other people carries Divine power, whether recognized as such or not. Divine power isn't metaphorical but literal, actually releasing calming chemicals in your brain. Study after study proves this. And Spirit does more than calm you; it heals you. It reverses entrenched patterns. It is nothing short of miraculous.

In my own life, I had an experience several years ago that, while not related to food, still demonstrates the power of exiting the isolation of your own suffering.

I had once flown on an airplane that lost an engine over the Pacific Ocean, and from that experience I developed a fear of takeoffs. It made no rational sense given that the engine on the plane hadn't quit upon takeoff, but my fear was what it was. Once a plane made its way above the clouds, I was fine. But until then, I was terrified.

I prayed for help, and then one day as I waited for takeoff, I found myself sitting next to a little boy who looked to be about seven or eight years old. He was sitting in his seat very straight and still, and I noticed that he seemed to be fighting back tears.

I looked at him and asked gently, "Are you alone, honey?" He nodded, looking straight ahead, his bottom lip trembling.

"Are you scared?" I asked. Again, he nodded.

"Would you like me to hold your hand?" I whispered into his ear. Again, he nodded.

At that point I went into full Mommy mode, gently talking to him as though I were reading him a nighttime story. Slowly, my voice lilting, I began to explain to him the process of takeoffs. "The pilot is turning on the engines now . . . that was the noise we just heard. . . . Now he's increasing the speed while we move down the runway . . . and at the right moment, when the pilot knows it is absolutely safe, the flaps on the wings will move—see them moving out there?—and that will create a lift and take the airplane into the sky! See? Isn't that beautiful? . . . The pilot is a really nice man, and he is totally in charge and knows exactly what to do to get the airplane into the sky and keep us all safe!"

Phew. He seemed relieved—and he wasn't the only one.

One might have thought I was an angel sent to comfort that little boy, but clearly he was an angel sent to comfort me. My fear of takeoffs ended that day. My pattern of anxiety was completely interrupted. In the midst of my fear, I reached out in love; then my fear was gone.

In both Katherine's case and mine, the miracle had manifested as a result of connecting compassionately with another person, extending if even for a moment beyond our own painful dramas to be of service to someone else.

Reaching out to other people is an integral part of your healing process, just as isolating is part of your disease. Isolating is a habit you formed long ago, and it has become a breeding ground for your compulsion. The fear-based mind needs only one moment to lure you into its lair, the secret place where no one else can enter. And at that point, you and food are off to the races.

The purpose of this lesson is to begin dismantling this pattern of isolation, reaching across the wall that separates you from others, and establishing a pattern of connection in the places where your heart has gone numb. This repatterning is your path to freedom.

You might be thinking that you have wonderful relationships with other people, and perhaps you do. Isolating, however, is a break in what might otherwise be a marvelous constellation of human relationships. You must develop the habit, at the moment when you isolate, to reach out for someone else. Connecting to another, you can stare down the doorman at the entrance to your alone zone.

The connection that saves you in such a moment could be an offer to help someone else, or simply an expression of your own vulnerability. It might be, "I know you're working two shifts on Saturday; would you like me to babysit your son?" Or it might be, "I'm having a hard time today. I just want to talk."

You may already be an extremely helpful person. Others would most probably look at you and call you anything *but* unloving. Disconnection is not just disconnection from the needs of others, but from your own needs as well. It is not overt unkindness, but merely disengagement. And in any moment of disconnection from love, you are prey to the pernicious delusion that you are hungry when in fact you are not.

Given that it takes only one moment to undo the value of months of right eating—starting you on a downward slide toward bingeing that can completely wreak havoc on both your psyche and your body—it is imperative that you see connecting more deeply with others as an ongoing necessity. Healing is a mind-set; it is a spiritual process whereby you leave behind an old way of being and fundamentally embrace a new relationship to life. In order to exit the alone zone, you must enter the connection zone. You must make your love, and also your needs, known to others.

Now make a list in your journal pages of various things you could do to increase your connection to other people. Sometimes it's an activity, while other times it's simply a shift in attitude that lets others get closer to you.

Two things occurred in my own life that helped me make such shifts. One was something that happened when I met a spiritual teacher from India several years ago. She had known me for maybe 15 minutes when she said simply, "Rigid and distant isn't working."

Her comment riveted me. This woman, who had never even met me before, had just given me the key to open the door I had locked against others. In seeking to defend myself, I had denied myself love. It didn't matter what the reason was for my disengagement—that I had begun to feel overwhelmed by the needs of others, or be hurt by their behavior, or had a need to retreat into a space of my own. What mattered is the personality characteristic I had developed as a defense against being hurt.

And what you defend against, you create. By trying to defend against being hurt by others, I was guaranteeing that I *would* be, for my rigid and distant behavior aroused criticism that hurt. Simply seeing this freed me to change.

The second example of something that melted a wall existing between myself and others was a comment once made by my daughter. She said something about how I acted a little coolly when people came up to have their books signed after my lectures. Nervously, I said to her, "Oh my God! I'm not polite? Am I not polite?" She responded, "No, Mommy, you're polite. But you're always the same. You're gracious, but you're not really that personal. You're nice to people, but you don't let anybody in."

I thought deeply about what my daughter said. I realized how much love I kept out of my life by keeping a certain professional wall up. That didn't mean I should refrain from having healthy boundaries, but it did mean that there was more love available to me than I was allowing myself to experience. And in any moment when we deny love, we trigger the original trauma that led us to isolate to begin with.

Developing a deeper connection to others is not something you can just check off your to-do list. You can't just *get it over with*. It is not a medicine you take and then just put back into the drawer once the sickness has passed. This issue—like everything about this course—involves a lifelong journey that once begun, never ends. It is a journey not simply into food recovery, but into a more light-filled life. It is a journey into the heart of love, toward others and toward yourself.

Any day devoted to love is a day when your craziness can't enter. It can knock at the door, but it can't come in. When you connect authentically with another person, the spell of your compulsion is broken. Just as a person in sub-zero temperatures knows better than to fall asleep, so it is incumbent upon you to be always on guard against the dangers of the Big Alone.

Daily, in your journal pages, note where you let others in that day and where you kept them out. Explore the places in your personality and in your lifestyle where you keep more space between yourself and others than you need to, where distance is not so much a healthy distance as an unhealthy one. Increased distance from others will lead to increased connection to food, as you run to the relationship that in a stressful moment feels like the one you can always count on.

In truth, you are in spiritual connection with people whether you turn away from them or not, because relationships occur on the level of the mind. Mystically, you are one with all living things. You cannot forget others and still remember who you are.

The simple act of connecting with other people will begin to break the chain that binds you. In any moment when you feel the void approaching, when you find yourself wanting to be alone so you can digest your poison—make a call, turn your car around, send an e-mail, make a move.

When you are grasping for starchy food like it is crack cocaine, do anything—the slightest thing—to connect with another person in a loving way. For in every righteous move you make toward others, you are making a move toward the experience of your own true self.

One instant at a time, one new response pattern at a time, one righteous human interaction at a time, you will lock the door of the ugly castle behind you, never to enter there again. And from the vantage point of where you go next—the clear outdoors where no obsessions rankle you—you will remember your hell with such gratitude for having been delivered from it.

And you will have a deep-seated desire to spend the rest of your life, whenever called, to help others make the same escape you did. In time, the psychic castle that housed your hell will be demolished and never house anyone again.

A recovering sufferer can recognize a sufferer, and a recovering sufferer intent on healing makes sure no sufferer in his or her path remains unloved. It's often just a knowing smile, a simple silent blessing, but it is a love that is sent from heaven to heal you both.

Remember to place your journal on the altar when you are done.

Reflection and Prayer

Close your eyes and relax into a holy space.

Ask Divine Mind to reveal the issues in your relationship that you need to address. Images will appear to you . . . relationship patterns where you could be more vulnerable or more helpful . . . places in your personality where you keep others at bay.

Ask to be shown how you appear to others, and how you can more fully express who you truly are. In this sacred space within your mind, you will be transformed from someone who avoids love to someone who embraces it . . . receives it . . . and is so filled up by it that nothing else is needed to make you feel full.

Dear God,
Please melt the walls
that separate me from others,
imprisoning me within myself.
Please heal my wounded places
and free my heart to love.
Help me connect to others
that I might isolate no more.
I know, dear God,
that when I am alone, I fear;
and when I fear, I self-destruct.
What I suffer now
and have suffered before,
dear God,
may I suffer no more.
Amen

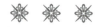

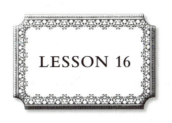

DISCIPLINE AND DISCIPLESHIP

You might be experiencing the "sunset effect" of an old self now, as the sun seems to be brightest in the moments just before it sets. The old self does not go quietly. She insists that you cannot live without her, she is your true self, and your entire world would fall apart were she not in charge. She does not sing merrily, "I'll see you around," as she wafts graciously out of the room. Rather, she most likely has hysterical fits in an effort to convince you that you cannot and will not ever be rid of her, so why try.

"Oh yeah?" she shrieks raucously. "You think you're going to break free, become healthy around food, lose weight, and just start over? Well, you're insane to think so! It will never work! I am your comfort; I am your strength; I am your power!" And then, of course, the only thing you can do is give in. Keep eating. Don't exercise. What's the point? And on and on. . . .

Her intensity, however, is but a cover for her frailty. In fact, she is so frail that she is fading away. Just as the Wicked Witch of the West in *The Wizard of Oz* simply melted when

Dorothy threw water on her, this mutant and predatory fragment of yourself is now dissolving into the nothingness out of which she emerged. As a nonreality, she cannot survive the waters of truth. As you embrace the vision of who you truly are, the false and illusionary being who has posed as you for all these years begins to disappear.

You have entered deeply into the process of your awakening, and in many ways you might find it as overwhelming as you feared it would be. The wild and out-of-control emotions that you've struggled so long to contain—creating, in so doing, your wild and out-of-control physical appetites— have all been stirred up.

Your detoxification process, both emotional and physical, is in full swing now. You may even be experiencing some chemical withdrawal as you let go of certain foods.

As an overeater, you've addressed the wildness of your emotional nature with what is ironically a very disciplined approach to life: *You will go eat now.* You have been disciplined, but disciplined by fear. What might have seemed to you or others like a complete lack of discipline on your part has actually been a strict adherence to an internal, dictatorial authority. The problem is that that internal authority is the voice of fear and compulsion instead of the voice of your true self.

As your mind realigns with its true self, your body will realign with *its* true self. Being a Divine creation, you know exactly what to do and how to be—on every level of your existence. Your bodily appetites are programmed naturally to follow the instructions of a Divine Intelligence. Your overeating, however, has been like a hacker that has reprogrammed your computer. What we're doing now is programming it back.

This reprogramming cannot be accomplished overnight. One aspect of your personality that has been damaged by your addictive tendencies is the ability to tolerate discomfort. When it comes to a compulsive urge to eat, you need it when you need it. *Results must occur immediately.* And now you are likely to exercise the same lack of impulse control and impose the same intolerance on your weight-loss process. *You want it and you want it now,* and if it doesn't happen by Thursday, then you might as well go back to your old habits, because obviously this doesn't work.

Now is a time to exercise discipline: not of your appetites, but of your thoughts. You know a lot about the discipline of fear; now it's time to learn about the discipline of love. Love is merciful, gentle, understanding, patient, forgiving, and kind. So you must be toward yourself as you go through this process.

No one needs to remind you of the many efforts you've made to lose weight in your past. It's not as though you haven't tried. Yet the same violence toward self that was displayed in the moment when you overate was then displayed when you fell off the wagon. *You're not good. You're a failure. You're weak. I hate you. Let's eat.*

Now look at what happens when you take a loving approach to weight loss. In a way, you're relearning how to feed yourself like a stroke victim might have to relearn how to speak or walk. Sometimes the smallest action represents the biggest step forward. A minimal improvement can be an important break from the past.

It might not seem like a big deal for someone else, but for you, it's extraordinary that you woke up one morning not obsessed with what you would eat today. For you, this represents a change, a pattern interruption, created in part by the work you've been doing with this course. And it builds on the musculature that will ultimately result in a new persona, new behavior, and new body. You deserve credit for this.

Please read that last sentence again. *You deserve credit for this.* Do not discount the significance of this change, for the slightest break in the chain of horror makes room for the beginning of a new chain—a chain of healthy thoughts and healthy appetites. This change, however small at first, must be affirmed, celebrated, and built upon—which it cannot be if you discount it. You are not in the habit of celebrating yourself when it comes to how you eat, and you owe it to yourself—and to this process—to learn to do it.

Conscious weight loss does not involve hating yourself; hatred is blasphemy, which means thinking that is contrary to the thoughts of God. That which is contrary to Divine Mind cannot possibly be your salvation, as your salvation lies in aligning with, not working against, the Divine. It is love and only love that will heal you. The miraculous change in perception here means going from hating how you have been, to loving the possibility of who you can now be.

You must choose the new you in order to become the new you. The issue here is not what you are running away *from*, but rather what you are running *toward*. You're not just rejecting what you don't want, but proactively claiming what you do.

The only way to break from your subconscious belief that eating is the source of your comfort is by building on your faith that *God* is the source of your comfort. Your relationship with the Divine is not just something to reluctantly embrace, as in "Okay, if I *have* to." It's the relationship that you most yearn for in your heart, whether you realize it or not. You can't break your dysfunctional habit of doing whatever the fear-mind commands except by building on your relationship with love. You must cultivate a passion for what you really, truly want. And what you really, truly want is love.

That is the meaning of discipleship, which obviously comes from the same root as the word *discipline*. Your problem is not *lack* of discipline, but rather *misplaced* discipline. Discipleship means disciplining yourself to serve the Divine.

The Divine is the source of your good, just as overeating is the source of your destruction. Serving the Divine leads to healing yourself, just as serving the fear-mind leads to hurting yourself. As you do these lessons, false comfort will give way to true comfort, and self-destruction will give way to self-nourishment and self-care. All of this is for one reason only: so you can better show up for love.

Isn't it extraordinary, if you think about it, how much energy human beings put into avoiding the idea that love is the answer? How many 800 numbers have you called, doctors have you seen, clinics have you been to, surgeries have you endured, seminars have you attended, fancy diets have you tried—all of which might have cost you resources of time and money you scarcely had—in an effort to try to get a plane into the air with what amounted to only one engine?

Love costs nothing. No time. No money. No effort, really. Yet the fear-mind, the mind that *is* your compulsion, would do anything to dissuade you from doing the one thing it knows would make it disappear in an instant. For the fear-mind is on its own quest for self-preservation. It doesn't mind your trying to lose weight, for it knows that without Divine help, you will be in its grip forever anyway. In fact, it loves to trip you up with one more diet that it knows you won't be able to stick to. According to *A Course in Miracles*, the dictate of the fear-mind, when it comes to love, will always be that you seek but do not find.

Begin to give more conscious attention to how your spiritual quest fits into your weight-loss efforts. Expand your thinking to a more soulful motivation for why you want to lose weight in the first place. Is it simply to look better? There is certainly nothing wrong with that, but of itself it doesn't attract spiritual support. As a bodily concern, it keeps your consciousness bound to the level of the body and is therefore nonmiraculous.

A more soulful motivation would be to make your body a container for greater light. When you dwell more lightly within your mind, you will dwell more lightly within your body. On both levels, your sense of well-being will increase. Your life choices will improve across the board, as both your mind and body develop more refined appetites. Your food choices will become more spiritual as you begin to see your body, and to feel your body, as part of a Divine matrix of love. That is the kind of miraculous impulse that attracts cosmic support. It aligns your desires with the larger drive toward greater life that is coded into the workings of the universe.

Your motivation then becomes not just about losing pounds, but about gaining enlightenment. Not the enlightenment of someone sitting under a tree in some far-off place in a remote part of the world, but rather the light-filled consciousness of someone who can wake up in the morning without the fear of an addictive lure—of being drawn against your will into the daze of inappropriate eating, of overly processed foods that you can't get enough of, and of chronic self-loathing.

You are getting there. The discomfort of emotional detox doesn't mean the process isn't working, but rather that it is. Do not let the ghosts of old emotions taunt you or deter you. It took more than a day to build the self-destructive mechanism that has caused you so much sorrow, and it takes more than a day to replace it with something new.

You are beginning to understand. One thought at a time, one healthier choice at a time, one moment-spent-free-of-the-monkey-on-your-back at a time, you are building the structure to contain the new you. And as a result, you will know joy. This process will bring far greater results than merely the pleasures of a lighter, healthier body. You will know the deep satisfaction of being in charge of your own life.

The subtlest changes in your thought-forms can radically transform the chemistry in your brain. While worldly voices might argue that only behavioral change produces "real change"—while spiritual change is hardly more than child's play—science itself is catching up to the most ancient wisdom regarding the powers of spirituality. The most prestigious academic institutions have conducted studies proving that those who are prayed for get out of intensive care units faster, that those who attend spiritual support groups survive longer after the diagnosis of a life-challenging illness, and so forth. Spirituality is more than simply an adjunct to what it *really* takes to lose weight.

If you are serious about wanting the power of spiritual forces to aid you in your weight loss, to provide at the very least your "second engine" to lift you miraculously above the forces of addiction and compulsion, then you must meet those forces with more than casual deference. You wouldn't want a worldly doctor to rush through his or her appointment with you; similarly, the Divine Physician needs you to spend a little more time at your appointments with Him.

Just as you wash your body daily, you need to purify your heart daily as well. When you neglect to pray and meditate on a regular basis—which means a daily basis—you leave your psychic door unlocked, and the thief *will* come in. Any day consciously and willingly given to God, praying that His guidance be with you and that you might be a conduit of love throughout the day, is a day when you are buffered from the otherwise active power of your fear-mind.

Your addictive impulses will be alert to the slightest forgetfulness on your part, and they will take advantage of the slightest opening ("I don't have time to pray and meditate today," "I don't need to reflect deeply on my behavior here;

I know what I'm doing!" "I'm angry for a good reason; this is not about forgiveness!") to rush back in with full-gale negative force.

The purpose of this lesson is (1) to establish the importance of "Spirit-time"—time taken every day to align your worldly self with your spiritual self, and (2) to help you establish this time as part of your daily routine. The most powerful aid to this is the practice of meditation.

True meditation is not mere relaxation, for it involves an actual shift in consciousness. There are many different meditation paths: Christian, Buddhist, or Jewish; the Workbook of *A Course in Miracles;* Transcendental, Vedic, or Vipassana Meditation; and more. A serious meditation practice is one of the most powerful ways to disconnect from your fear-mind and its fearful dictates.

Too much attention to the earth plane creates undue stress on the body. Meditation frees the mind from its attachment to the body, thus freeing the body to right itself. As you set your mind free of physical attachments for a period of time each day, you improve your relationship to the physical world.

Some people claim they don't have time to meditate. But meditation *slows down time.* And in slowing down time, you slow down and rebalance your nervous system. Stress leads to frenetic energy, and frenetic energy leads to impulsive behavior. Meditation, by reducing stress, brings calm to both your body and your mind.

Meditation is like a sealant, protecting your devotional energy so the light cannot slip out and the darkness cannot enter. Emotionally, you will be lifted higher and higher, gaining a more and more consistent sense of joy. With that, the gravitational lure of self-destructive urges will decrease and ultimately cease.

But meditation is more than lighting a candle and breathing deeply; it is more than walking through the woods or speaking a beautiful intention. I've heard many people say, "I *do* meditate. I meditate by journaling, by reading inspirational literature, by spending quiet time alone." All those things are good—indeed, they've been recommended as a part of this course. But they are relaxation, inspiration, and contemplation; they are *not* of themselves meditation. Meditation is something deeper, something that actually changes your brain waves. And for that you need a serious meditation practice.

There is a meditation path that will work for you, and you might even know what it is already. Whether or not you will avail yourself of this medicine of the gods is completely up to you.

Just remember that meditation is so powerful that the fear-mind will tell you anything to make you believe it isn't powerful, or it isn't for you, or you just don't have time to do it. "I don't know how to meditate." (But you could learn.) "I tried meditation, but I couldn't stick with it." (Change "couldn't" to "didn't.") It is your choice, of course, which voice in your head to listen to, which voice to believe, and most important of all, which voice to act on.

If you have a meditation practice, then nothing could be more important to transforming your relationship to food than that you *do* it. And if you do not have a meditation practice but pray to be shown one, then books or flyers that lead to one that is best for you will begin to fall at your feet.

Addiction is a spiritual disease; prayer and meditation boost the spiritual immune system. You are not fighting the disease; you are simply opening your mind to so much truth that the diseased condition cannot dwell there. Your goal is for the light to seep into the deepest recesses of your subconscious mind, erasing old patterns and releasing your mind to new ones.

Overeating is an act of hysteria, and meditation is the most powerful antidote to hysteria. Hysteria occurs when you lose your conscious connection with the naturally ordered universe, and in that traumatic moment try to absorb the shock of cosmic disorder by grabbing for a bite-size piece of comfort. Enough has been said of your separation from love; our focus now is on your return to it.

You have had moments, surely, when love has prevailed and you were not tormented by your compulsion. You have had moments when you sailed through your kitchen and felt no insane need to eat inappropriately. The problem is that the insanity has always returned, sometimes when you would least expect it. Various efforts have given you temporary surcease from the overwhelming compulsion to reenact your pattern, but none have totally *stopped* the pattern. Only the hand of God can do that.

Thus, this entire situation is an invitation to discipleship. It's time to give Him *all* of your time and *all* of your days and *all* of your thoughts. Your mind is holy, yet you must stand on that knowledge. You must actively embrace the truth in order to receive its blessing. For any moment not given to love will be used by fear as a breeding ground for its own purposes. Choose love, so fear will no longer be able to choose you.

Discipleship is a sacred marriage. Only the arms of God can truly hold you and keep you and protect you from all harm. Once you've experienced the embrace of your Divine Beloved, perhaps you will choose to commit to Him. You will promise to cleave to Him and "forsake all others." Having made this commitment, you will break off your relationship with the tyrant of compulsion that has masqueraded as your lover. And that is what discipleship is: a total commitment that leaves no room for anything else.

Discipleship is much, much more than a sometimes thing; it's an effort to totally immerse yourself in the light of love. And this will do more than just transform your eating. It will transform your entire life.

Take anything that symbolizes the meditation path that calls to you—from the phone number of a meditation teacher you have heard about but not yet called, to the Workbook of *A Course in Miracles,* to a set of prayer beads—and place it on your altar for consecration to the Divine.

Reflection and Prayer

Close your eyes and relax into your sacred place. See yourself in your inner temple, a beautiful and holy room. See yourself lying in the center of it, on a large white slab. The slab looks like cold marble—but when you lie down, it feels like warm, soft pillows.

Now see the Divine Physician standing above you with His hands over your body. The Divine being is drawing from your body all the energy that does not belong there, both physical and nonphysical. Breathe deeply into this image and allow it to be real for you. Such imagery is no idle fantasy. Spirit is always present, not just metaphorically but literally.

Now continue with an exercise from *A Course in Miracles.* With your eyes closed, say slowly to yourself, "Into His presence would I enter now." Repeat the sentence over and over to yourself as you fall more and more deeply into a meditative state. Allow yourself a minimum of five minutes doing this.

As you practice this exercise, you will sense its meaning more and more as time goes by. It will help prepare you for a formal meditation practice, and open your mind to absorb its power.

Dear God,
Thank You for the things that I have seen.
When on the mountaintop, I have felt such joy.
Please send angels
to lift me up
and always hold me tenderly.
Do not let insanity take hold of me,
but enlighten me that I might be free.
Place my feet on a higher path
and show me how to walk in love,
that I might find my way.
Amen

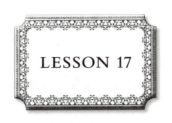

FORGIVE YOURSELF
AND OTHERS

According to *A Course in Miracles,* all thought creates form on some level. If your "weighty thinking" does not change, then even if you lose weight, you'll retain an overwhelming subconscious urge to gain it back. It's less important how quickly you lose weight, and more important how *holistically* you lose weight; you want your mind, your emotions, and your body to *all* "lose weight." Weight that disappears from your body but not from your soul is simply recycling outward for a while, but is almost certain to return. It's self-defeating, therefore, to struggle to drop excess weight unless you are also willing to drop the thought-forms that initially produced it and now hold it in place.

Judgment and blame are the weightiest thoughts of all, as they lack love. They are products of the fear-mind, representing the densest energy in the universe—the perception of someone's guilt. Learning to forgive both yourself and others is the greatest gift you can give yourself on your path to conscious weight loss.

Compulsive eating separates you from others, and forgiveness heals the separation. Once again, you might have wonderful connections with people, but any breakage at all is a place where the devil can get in. Unless you address your relationship issues themselves, then they will always lurk in the back of your mind, able to trip the addictive switch back to ON at any time.

In order to deal with your weight loss from a holistic perspective, you must address your issues with relationships as seriously as you address your issues with food. Losing weight will not of itself heal your relationships, but healing your relationships will help you lose weight.

Forgiveness is critical, as we all make little as well as big mistakes, and little as well as big judgments. Cultivating a forgiving attitude softens the edges of human contact. It's an aspect of what is called the Atonement, or the correction of our perceptions from fear back to love. The purpose of this lesson is to atone for any lack of forgiveness on your part, releasing excess weight that lies heavy on your heart.

There are two basic filters through which to view all things: the filter of the body, and the filter of the spirit. To the extent that you view your life only through the body's filter, you are bound to the body in a way that does not serve you. Being bound to the body, you are at the effect of the body's appetites, whether they are healthy or dysfunctional. But when your eyes are lifted, giving you the capacity to see beyond the body to the realm of your spirit, you're given power over your body that otherwise you do not have. Dwelling lightly within your body, your body becomes light.

And how do you do that? How do you see *beyond* the body? You do it by being willing to extend your focus beyond the dramas of the material plane, remembering that beyond this drama there is the truer truth of who we all are.

Yes, a friend might have said something cruel to you— but in her heart, she's simply lost and lonely like everyone else. Your friend does love you; she was just disconnected from her love at the moment when she made that hurtful comment.

No matter what happens to you, you have a choice as to how to interpret it. You will make that choice—consciously or subconsciously. You can focus on the body's drama—your friend's unkind words, her mistake, her betrayal. But if you do, you won't be able to escape the emotional experience of being at the effect of her words.

By choosing to focus on the material drama, particularly the drama of guilt, you increase your attachment to the material plane and thus your vulnerability to its dysfunctions. You forgive because you wish to stay above the dramas of the material world, particularly the drama of your compulsion.

You can choose to focus on the innocence in your friend—on her Divine reality that is beyond, and truer, than her bodily self. All of us are made of love, yet all of us make mistakes. In detaching from an overemphasis on someone else's mistakes, you detach from an overemphasis on your own. As you reach across the wall of separateness—and there is no wall thicker than the wall of judgment—then the wall comes down. That is the miracle of forgiveness.

Forgiveness is like preventive medicine. It cancels out the lie at the center of the fear-mind, robbing it of its ability to hurt you. The fear-mind jams your personal radar system, disconnecting you from Divine Mind and leading you toward thoughts and behaviors that destroy your inner peace. It tells you that you are less than perfect, tearing you from the memory of your Divine self. From there, it's easy to convince you that no one else is Divinely perfect either.

Fear-mind's mantra is: *Guilt, guilt, and more guilt.* It casts you into judgmental consciousness—whether judgment of yourself or others—dooming you to an emotional seesaw ride between love and fear. That seesaw is emotionally unstable, and is one of the biggest threats to your food sobriety.

The fear-mind doesn't have to convince you to eat excessively so much as it just has to convince you that someone is guilty, for the perception of guilt is enough to throw you out of your right mind and thus into your disease. An attitude of forgiveness takes you off—or keeps you off—the seesaw.

Forgiveness is a selective remembering. It is a conscious choice to focus on someone's innocence instead of his or her mistakes. In common parlance, it usually amounts to simply cutting people more slack. This serves *you*. Judgment and blame put stress on the body of whoever is doing the judging and blaming, and stress is the time bomb at the center of your addictive urge.

It is in "staying above" the drama of the body that you dwell more harmoniously within it. Your body was not created to bear the burden of your overattachment to it, but was created as a container for the light of your spirit. It will more easily remember how to function perfectly when you remember the perfection in everyone.

Forgiveness is hugely powerful yet often resisted fiercely. A young man I knew in an AIDS support group years ago once asked me, "Do I really have to forgive *everybody?*" To which I responded, "Well, I don't know . . . do you have the flu, or do you have AIDS? Because if you only have the flu, then, heck, just forgive a few people . . . but if you have AIDS, then, yes, try to forgive everybody!"

You certainly wouldn't ask a doctor, "Do I really have to take *all* the medicine? Take the *entire round* of chemo? Can't I just do *some* of it?" Nor would you say, "Doc, can I just take the medicine when I feel bad?" No, medicine is medicine. And you respect it enough to take the amount you need.

Forgiveness is more than just a good thing. It is key to right living and thus to your healing—not just to be applied every once in a while, but to be aimed for as a constant. None but enlightened masters achieve forgiveness all the time, but the effort itself keeps the arrows of attack at bay. Holding on to judgment, blame, attack, defense, victimization, and so forth are absolutely attacks on yourself. And you attack yourself with food.

As you forgive others, you begin to forgive yourself. As you stop focusing on their mistakes, you will stop punishing yourself for your own. Your ability to release what you think of as the sins of others will free you to release yourself, putting down that particular weapon with which you punish yourself so savagely.

Forgiveness releases the past to Divine correction and the future to new possibilities. Whatever it was that happened to you, it is *over*. It happened in the past; in the present, it does not exist unless you bring it with you. Nothing anyone has ever done to you has permanent effects unless you hold on to it permanently.

Your first task with this lesson is to identify those whom you have not forgiven. Know that even the slightest annoyance with someone is enough to throw your system out of Divine right order. Do not just focus here on the people who have deeply betrayed or wounded you; think about even those who, for reasons that are seemingly small, still tempt you to withhold your love from them. For wherever you withhold your love, you deflect your miracle.

Use your journal pages to list the names of all people whom, in your heart, you know you still judge. They can range from a parent to a political figure. Your anger at them, not who they are or what they have done, is what matters. When a name occurs to you, write it down, along with the feelings you associate with that person—anger, hurt, betrayal, contempt, fear, and so forth. Explore your feelings as deeply as you can, and try not to rush through the process. After you've explored your lack of forgiveness, write down these words: "I am willing to see this person differently." Write that sentence three times, as it is very important.

Painful circumstances can form a veil over your eyes, making it difficult to appreciate others' Divine innocence when their behavior was so contrary to it. By expressing a willingness to see them differently, you call on the power of Divine Mind. You'll receive Divine help as long as you're *willing* to forgive. You'll receive a reminder of who those people really are, beyond the things you don't like about them. Sometimes all you need is a tweak in consciousness— a reminder that you're blaming someone for something that you yourself do all the time, perhaps—and sometimes you need otherwordly help in lifting a burden otherwise too hard to bear.

From abandoned spouses to victims of the Holocaust, I've heard of miraculous changes in the hearts of those who prayed for such help and received it. Sometimes forgiveness is a small thing, and sometimes it is huge. Yet forgiveness isn't simply a gift you give someone else; it is a gift you give yourself. The density and pain of your negative feelings toward anyone is a weight you carry. And you are learning to live a lighter life.

This awakening involves realizing the light in others and also the light in you. Sometimes the person you most need to forgive is yourself. All of us are human, and most of us have done something we regret. We all carry walls in front of our heart, and we all feel guilt when we have wronged someone.

Looking at your own transgressions and atoning for them is an important part of your healing. For whether it's conscious or not, any guilt you carry has made you feel on a deep level that you deserve punishment. And overeating is one of the ways in which you have punished yourself. Let's get the trial started so we can get you acquitted right away.

Write down the names of everyone you think you've wronged, every mistake you feel you've made, every regret you still carry. Apologize in your heart for any transgression toward others or toward yourself. Look at each name or event, then prayerfully release it into the hands of God. Say aloud, to yourself or to the memory of anyone to whom you owe an apology: "I am sorry."

It's tempting to ignore or minimize old transgressions, thinking, *Oh well, it was a long time ago. . . .* As intent as the fear-mind is at monitoring the wrongs of others, it is exceptionally good at getting you to overlook your own. Someone might have hurt you 15 years ago and you're still talking about it—but *you* might have hurt *someone else* 15 years ago and haven't thought about it for the last 14. But until an unloving energy is acknowledged and atoned for, it remains an active toxin poisoning your life.

Amends that are 20 years late are still amends that need to be made. If you hurt other people, then even if they don't consciously remember what you did to them, they carry the pain within their cells. And so do you. On the level of spirit, we are all one, and what you have done to hurt someone else is a hurt you carry within yourself.

It can be very humbling to reach out and apologize. It can be embarrassing at first to admit your own mistake. Yet such moments as these are moments of mastery, freeing you from the prison of your own insanity. You have atoned for your error, and you are free to begin again.

Your willingness to make amends to those you hurt in the past carries with it more power than a thousand diet plans. The fear-mind is a false sense of oneself as an isolated and separate human being. Whenever you make amends for having harmed another, you acknowledge that you are not separate—that there is more to life than your own drama. You acknowledge that another person's experience is as important as your own, and you realize that by hurting someone else, you have hurt yourself.

The shift in your thinking—from ignoring your own transgressions to admitting them and being willing to make amends where appropriate—is a miracle that produces practical consequences in your life. As you reach across the wall of separateness, the wall begins to come down.

The fear-mind would argue that forgiveness has nothing to do with your weight or with your food issues, but if anything should be clear by now, it's that the fear-mind lies. You're beginning to realize that underlying every problem in your life is a false sense of separation, between you and others and between you and your true self.

Any path to permanent weight loss addresses your sense of isolation and the despair it spawns. Keeping love at bay, you've kept the healed and peaceful you at bay. In forgiving others, you're finally free to experience the joy of feeling close to them—with no wall between you necessary. And in forgiving yourself, you realize you deserve to look as beautiful on the outside as you've remembered, at last, that you are beautiful within.

Reflection and Prayer

Do this meditation regarding any and every person from whom you are separated by unforgiving thoughts or feelings.

Take a deep breath and close your eyes.

Now see with your inner eye a vision of that person standing on the left side of your mind. See his or her body, clothes, mannerisms, and way of being in the world. Now see a great light in the middle of that person's heart, spreading to cover every cell of the body and extending outward beyond the flesh and into infinity. Watch as the light becomes so bright that his or her body begins to fade into shadow.

Now gently see a vision of your own body on the right side of your inner vision. Here, too, see your mannerisms, your clothes, your way of being in the world. And see the same Divine light in the area of your own heart, moving outward to cover every cell of your body and extending into infinity beyond the confines of your flesh. Watch as the light grows so bright that your body begins to fade into shadow.

Now slowly move your inner eye to the middle of your field of vision, where the light from deep within the other person and the light from deep within you begin to merge. Simply look, and allow yourself to witness this Divine oneness. *The joining that you see here is the reality of love.*

Spend as much time as you can with this vision each time you do it, hopefully a minimum of five minutes. It carries the power of a holy truth impressed on your subconscious mind.

Do this meditation again, making both people your own self. Pray for a Divine reconciliation between who you've been and who you really are. Rest deeply into these images, and allow the illumination to cast all darkness from your mind. This is the highest reconciliation of all: you with the real you.

Dear God,
Please teach me to forgive
myself and others.
Remove the walls
that keep love out,
behind which I am prisoner.
Heal my guilt
and remove my anger,
that I might be reborn.
Make gentle my heart
and strong my spirit
and show me how to love.
Amen

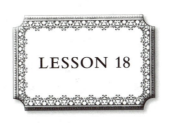

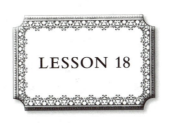

LESSON 18

HONOR
THE PROCESS

There's a possibility that you're sick of this course by now. You might not have even made it to this point; you might just be picking up the book, opening it wherever, and simply happen to be reading this. You might be thinking that it's all too hard, too confronting, or even a bunch of nonsense. You might not have seen any real changes on your scale or in your mirror yet, and have decided that by Lesson 18 you should be having *some* success. Clearly this is not a miracle, and you might as well just forget it.

See how the fear-mind works?

That's how the fear-mind works in *everyone*. For one person, she shouldn't even try to finish writing that novel, because she never will and she's not a good writer anyway—according to the fear-mind. For another, he shouldn't even bother going to that interview because he's been out of circulation too long, and companies are only hiring younger people anyway—according to the fear-mind. For another, she shouldn't even try to dress up and look nice, because she's not attractive anyway—according to the fear-mind.

The fear-mind lives in everyone, but it speaks differently to all of us. To you, it just happens to be obsessed with your weight, because you are.

Learning to live with the common disappointments and failures of the human experience—particularly with how the fear-mind interprets them—is part of your spiritual mastery.

Mastery doesn't mean you get to the point where nothing ever goes wrong; it means you get to the point where you can endure and transform what's wrong. Mastery means you rise up more often than you sink in life, not because in you there is no undertow, but because you've learned to swim well. You're spiritually strong and in shape. You've developed your attitudinal muscles, and they can carry you when you're feeling the gravitational pull of whatever your temptation might be.

Mastery is not superhuman, but deeply human; embracing rather than resisting the realization that on certain days you'll feel like master of nothing and slave to lots of things. Do not let the fact that you have fallen off the wagon, are falling off the wagon, haven't lost any weight yet, can't stand to do the lessons, or still feel like a big fat loser deter you. This is all part of the process. And your success is guaranteed.

Now the fear-mind gets really activated. "What do you *mean*, my success is *guaranteed?!* Guaranteed by *whom?*" Almost as in, how dare I say that? But it's my faith—and you can lean on mine if you wish—that God will wipe away every tear, that He will outwit all self-hatred, and that in Him is the victory as soon as we give to Him the fight.

None of that means that every day will be a happy one. Serious weight loss is a deeply transformative experience; you're breaking a chain that has held you tight for a very long time, and it's only reasonable to expect that some days will be harder than others. This is not just a physical battle; it is a spiritual battle. The fear-mind has robbed you of your self-control . . . and God is taking it back.

Winston Churchill famously told British troops during World War II: "Now this is not the end. It is not even the beginning of the end. But it is, perhaps, the end of the beginning." This course is not something that is all over in 21 lessons. It is a means to weight loss and also weight-loss maintenance. What it lays out is not a goal so much as a process by which the goal will be achieved. You do not do it solely to lose weight, but in order to become the most shining expression of who you are as a human being.

If your only goal is to lose weight, then hopefully you will do so, but you'll still be left with other issues to deal with that cannot be denied. Issues in your life seemingly unrelated to weight have accumulated around your relationship to food.

In any moment when you feel overwhelmed by a passion to overeat, remember that the passion itself is not the problem. The problem is that in a moment of insane eating, your passion for life is displaced onto something that doesn't give you life but rather sucks life from you. This course is building a detour, redirecting your passion away from food and back to God.

To which the fear-mind says, "Screw you. I won't do it." Just want to make sure you realize that. The mind cannot serve two masters, and never in your life has the choice between the two been so clear. In any moment, you are either host to God or hostage to the fear-mind. It is not enough to say no to a life of fear; you must say yes to a life of love. As long as you try to stay neutral, you will overeat.

Weight is your crucible. It's the place where you experience the final spiritual battle between the forces of fear and the forces of love—in psychological terms, between dysfunctional appetites and healthy impulses. The decision you are making is not just whether you'll rise *from* the hell of your compulsion, but whether you'll rise *into* the heaven of all the joy-filled possibilities that await you. The fear-mind leads to suffering as sure as Divine Mind leads to joy. The various ways people anesthetize themselves today—whether through substances or pharmaceuticals—is a wail from the deep: "Please don't make me have to choose."

But choose you must, for the zone of false neutrality has become increasingly unsustainable for you. You *will* see the light of your true being, and your only choice is what path you take to get there. So merciful is the universe that even a path of darkness includes a way back to light. Peacock feathers are made by peacocks eating and then digesting thorns. You have been eating the thorns of addiction and compulsion for a very long time; now you're spiritually digesting them, inwardly preparing for their transformation from something ugly to something beautiful.

There is a line in the New Testament that states: "What man intends for evil, God intends for good." Divine Mind will not simply cast out your compulsion; it will use it to take you higher than if you had never experienced such depths. You will emerge from this experience no longer compulsive about food, yes. But you will also emerge filled with a light that you can only cast because you digested such darkness. Such is the greatness of God.

Do not be emotionally defeated by whatever time it takes for old patterns to transform. Do not look to the mirror for confirmation of your faith. When a woman is first pregnant, the outer eye cannot see it, but it will in time. Your mirror can show changes in your body, but it does not show changes in your mind. On any given day, the mirror shows you what your thinking was yesterday, but it's what's happening in your heart today that creates what your life will be tomorrow. You decrease your body weight by expanding your mind.

A spiritual process is not a quick fix; it is a miracle imprinted on you by Divine Mind. It is help that is brought to you from beyond this world. It is nothing that you your-self can just "make happen," but you can honor the mysteri-ous process by which it does.

To the fear-mind, the very concept of spiritual mystery—particularly related to weight loss—seems ridiculous. The fear-mind is attached to the body, and wants to make sure that you are attached to it, too. If the body's eyes don't reg-ister improvement in your weight, the fear-mind will say, "See? See?" And if the body's eyes do register improvement, the fear-mind will say, "Ah! But it will not last!"

What could be a more worthy endeavor than giving time every morning and evening to quieting the fear-mind? To listening instead to the voice for God? You won't feel over-whelmed by the void once you fill it with the Divine.

It does not matter how long it takes. It does not matter how many times you might have succeeded then failed, suc-ceeded then failed. Your direction is sure at last, for you have given it over to a Divine authority.

Your motivation is different now, and that will make all the difference: you are on a quest to find the holy grail of the authentic you. You are climbing above the turbulence of your compulsive eating not only because you want to lose weight, but because you want the serenity found only at higher altitudes. Up there, there will be no monkey on your back, for monkeys cannot live that high.

Every time you get it right—no matter how large or small your victory—you are asserting your spiritual power and regaining authority over your life. Whether it's turning away from ice cream or putting on your gym shoes when you absolutely don't feel like it, you are winning.

You are experiencing the force of your true self—the self that's healing, that's transforming, that's rising above, that's becoming sober around food. The positive act was an example of the real you blazing the way, if even for a moment, through the veils of compulsion into full embodiment. The anti-gravitational pull of grace is luring you upward.

And for that, we rejoice. One moment of truth—and the real you *is* truth—reprograms a thousand years of lies. A new condition is making its way into your experience. Even the slightest right-minded thought or action—"I am passing by the refrigerator, but I am choosing not to open it"; "I do not numb myself with overly processed foods, because I choose to be more fully available to my life"; "My body is a holy temple, and I want to feed it healthy and nourishing food"; "I am shining and radiant in spirit and my body reflects that"—bolsters the process by which new appetites and new patterns of behavior are being formed.

Try your best to be patient during this process. Support yourself by avoiding situations that would be likely to tempt you into addictive behavior. You deserve the same support from yourself that you would give any friend or family member whom you love.

Be supportive enough of yourself to say "No" when the most powerful move would be to say "No." Not only to avoid the food, but to affirm the most powerful you. "No, I will not go over to the dessert table. No, I will not go out tonight because I know that group will just sit around eating. No, I will not buy that bag of chocolate."

And be supportive enough of yourself to say "Yes" when the most powerful move would be to say "Yes." "Yes, I will check out kale salad even though I've never eaten that kind of food before. Yes, I will pick up that yoga video today. Yes, I will take a walk in the park and allow my body to feel more healthy and productive." Even the smallest efforts can have huge effects.

Some of those effects go way beyond weight loss, influencing your thinking about other things as well. For instance, this situation has given you an opportunity to realize more fully the suffering that many people go through every day of their lives. Your own efforts at transformation have made you understand more deeply both the pain as well as the redemptive opportunities of the human race. Through your suffering, you will come to have real wisdom; and through your wisdom, you will come to know joy.

But are you ready for joy, really? Are you ready to be the person who does not suffer from this compulsion? Who does not obsess about food? Who does not act against your own self-interest in such a pernicious way? Are you ready to let go of not only the behavior of overeating, but also the very consciousness of the person who overeats? Are you ready for food to no longer even be a *big deal* in your life? Are you ready to be spiritually born anew into the light of your true being as a child of the Divine, over whom such darkness as food compulsion holds no sway? Are you ready to let go of the psychological and emotional habits, not just the physical ones, that have fueled your compulsion?

These are the questions life puts in front of you now. If your answer to all of them is a passionate yes, then you are on the path to rebirth. And even if it's a weary yes, your way forward is guaranteed.

Now your task is to write a letter. It's like a Dear John letter to the imposter who's been masquerading as you, the person who sneaks into the kitchen to eat whatever she can find, who gets into the car to scour the neighborhood for whatever is open so she can get some food, who cannot control herself when food is present in the room, who hides in big clothes and cannot bear the sight of the mirror. She isn't you; she's just an illusion of you who has snuck her way into your three-dimensional reality and will leave the instant you command her to. When Jesus said, "Satan, get thee behind me," that's what he meant.

Even in a moment when you've given in and begun to overeat, realizing with horror that you're headed down that dark and slippery slope, don't despair. When you hear your fear-mind arguing, "Well, I already ate the cake, so I may as well go for the M&M's. Why bother to stop now? I already messed up, so I may as well continue," own your power and command her to leave.

Refusal to eat the first bite of cake is not your only chance for a moment of power. It's just as significant when, having eaten the cake already, you can refuse the second piece, or the entire bag of M&M's sitting in the cabinet. Any point of the process is a moment of power, if it's a moment of conscious choice on behalf of your sane and self-loving self.

Say out loud: "In the name of God, I command that you leave." You don't have to believe me that this works; you will find out for yourself.

The letter you now write is both a command and a good-bye. It is a leave-taking, a statement of independence from a master you will no longer allow to enslave you, and with whom you no longer agree to conspire. Remember that the letter, once written, belongs on your altar.

The letter includes three parts:

1. Why I allowed you to live in me, and the ways that I said yes to you:

Example: *As much as I hated you, you were something I could hide behind. I didn't have to really show up for my life, because I always had an excuse why this or* *that wasn't a real option for me. In hiding behind you, I didn't have to face my fear of being skinny and beautiful and really participating in life.*

2. Why I no longer need you, and what I have come to realize:

Example: *I have learned that there is strength within me that I never knew I had. I have realized that there is a Divine spirit in me, and I serve no one by refusing it. It is a gift from God and it is humble, not arrogant, to live in this spirit. I am a child of a Divine Creator, and it is my responsibility to the universe, not just a gift to myself, to receive His spirit and allow it to direct me in everything I do.*

3. What I say to you now, through the authority of Divine Mind:

Example: *What we had is over. In the name of God, I command you to release me. In the name of God, I command you to depart. In the name of God, the door shall be sealed behind you. And so it is.*

Your letter is an adjunct to a paragraph from my book *A Return to Love,* which has resonated with many people seeking to repudiate their weaknesses and embrace their God-given strengths:

Our deepest fear is not that we are inadequate. Our deepest fear is that we are powerful beyond measure. It is our light, not our darkness, that most frightens us. We ask ourselves, who am I to be brilliant, gorgeous, talented, fabulous? Actually, who are you *not* to be? You are a child of God. Your playing small does not serve the world. There is nothing enlightened about shrinking so that other people won't feel insecure around you. We are all meant to shine, as children do. We were born to make manifest the glory of God that is within us. It's not just in some of us; it's in everyone. And as we let our own light shine, we unconsciously give other people permission to do the same. As we are liberated from our own fear, our presence automatically liberates others.

You are not yet, perhaps, fully liberated from your own fear. But you are getting there. Within the holiness of your own mind, you're beginning to see the outlines of a you who has left this hell behind her. Consider the mere idea of her existence; breathe in the thought; embrace the possibility. And she will begin to take shape.

The healed you is not an expression of a "managed" situation, but rather of a truly transformed one. She does not yet have deep roots within your nervous system, but she has roots within your soul. As the memory of the real you, she is a creation of the Divine. And what is Divinely created cannot be uncreated. The true you, free of all torment related to food, lives already in the realm of Divine Mind and is waiting for your permission to be born into the world.

I join with you in absolute conviction that she *will* be born. And she embodies something far more glorious than merely a healthy relationship to food. She delivers a peace that only love can bestow.

During this time of gestation, have faith in what is happening inside you. Do not let appearances fool you. Do not look at your flesh and wince. Do not look at it and give in to self-loathing. Yes, old flesh undoubtedly remains, but its cause is fading even as you read this. Looking at your body, realize that it is a changeable condition. Your flesh has merely responded to your mind. Now celebrate that you are *changing* your mind.

The womb of your consciousness has been impregnated with a Divine idea: the thought that a permanently freer, more perfect you is possible. This impregnation is a mystery into which your soul must enter, as you allow to occur within you a miraculous process of death and rebirth. The old you, the obsessive you—the one who carries all the patterns of your pain—will now cease to exist.

Who you used to be, you will be no longer—and who you were created to be will now shine forth. She is taking form inside a sacred place—the realm of infinite possibility that lives inside your heart. Turn there and you will find her. She is waiting for you. And she will appear in the twinkling of an eye.

Reflection and Prayer

Close your eyes and relax into a meditative space.

On the left side of your mind, see yourself as you manifest addictively. See yourself behaving compulsively. Now, on the right side of your mind, see the real you, the free you, the sober you, the radiant you. See cords of darkness and dysfunction, thick and ugly, which connect the real you to your addictive self.

Now see an angel, sent by God, walk up to the cords with a scissors of light. Watch carefully as the angel *cuts the cords*. The cords are dark and gnarly, yet the Divine scissors cuts right through them. See them drop to the floor and sink below the surface of the ground, disappearing for all time. Hear angels singing in the background. Bear witness to whatever happens now, and give thanks that you are free.

Dear God,
I am ready to die to whom I used to be,
and be born to whom I wish to be.
But of myself I can do neither.
Transform me at the deepest levels,
that I might suffer no more
the pain of unreality.
Impregnate my soul with the seed
of my true self,
that I might know joy and peace at last.
Amen

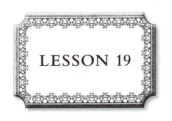

BIRTHING WHO
YOU REALLY ARE

Losing weight is either a managed condition or a miracle. If it's a managed condition, then that's great, but it rests on unstable moorings. If it's a miracle, it rests on God.

There's little point in trying to bring forth a thinner you, unless it's a thinner you with a fairly good chance of *remaining* a thinner you. Otherwise, you end up back in that corner of hell where your soul cries out in horror, "I can't believe I did this again . . ."

You need, then, more than just weight loss. You need a miracle. When you're in the throes of an addictive impulse, however, you make yourself unavailable to receive one. In order to birth the miracle of a new you, you must be open to the love that pierces your invisible shield.

A miracle is a shift in perception from fear to love, creating breakthroughs in your experience by creating breakthroughs in your mind. Much of the work involved in this course has been an inquiry into what it is, exactly, that you fear . . . particularly as it relates to other people. This lesson involves identifying any fear you might harbor toward an aspect of yourself: the possible new you.

The universe, being the handwriting of God, is a continuous flow of love. Yet the fear-mind seeks to block that love just as continuously as Spirit pours it forth. It would keep you locked in repetitive patterns that prevent you from becoming who you are capable of being. As long as your mind is in service to fear, you are bound to your past. Only in serving love are you free to move forward into a new and truly different future.

Of course you don't consciously serve fear. The problem is that fear permeates the ethers of the world in which you live, and fear breeds the addictive impulse. The fear-mind knows that if *you* get to fully live, then it has to die. It is literally fighting for its life, as are you.

Yet you cannot take on the fear-mind directly. You don't get rid of it by fighting it, but only by transcending it; not by attacking it, but by replacing it. You have spent much of your life saying no to your addiction, but the key to your freedom lies in saying yes to the possible you. The purpose of this lesson is to remove any barriers you still hold that are keeping you from becoming your truest self.

To become the truest you, you must actively embrace the truest you. But this you cannot do if you are ambivalent about this aspect of yourself, or even neutral toward her. In the absence of your heartfelt invitation, she cannot come. This future you—one who lives the highest manifestation of your Divine potential—cannot pierce the fear-mind's veil and simply come toward you. It is your choice—the choice of the current you—whether or not to remove the veil and move toward her. The only way to give her birth into the world is by loving her with all your heart.

It's a big decision whether or not to embrace her, for in doing so you will become one with her. And for this, you must be ready. You know in your heart that in becoming her, you will lose some aspects of your current personality.

Your identity has been wrapped up with being who you are now, even though you are filled with certain aspects of fear and self-loathing. When you look at your resistance, you can begin to remove it. When you look at your fear, you can begin to surrender it. That which is possible will only become probable when and if it is beckoned by love.

And who is the new you? First of all, she loves you completely—is that true of who you are now? She is comfortable in your body—is that true of who you are now? She has a healthy relationship with food—is that true of who you are now? She thinks you're beautiful—is that true of who you are now? It's important—in fact, it's necessary—to realize these gaps in your alignment with your truest self, for then you can give them to Divine Mind for healing. If you do not surrender them, then you might have described them but you will not have removed them. These gaps are the thinnest membrane, really. They are merely thoughts. But there is no wall more intractable than a wall of fearful thoughts, just as there is nothing that can remove the wall more completely than thoughts of love.

Now let's face your biggest fear: that of giving birth to a new you. It's not your fear of being fat, but your fear of being thin—your fear of being free, your fear of being extraordinary, your fear of being your most joyful self. For who, then, will you be? What will you do with yourself? Who will love you? Who will reject you? What will you do when people approach you with the vibes of sexual attraction? What will people say about you? How will you dress? Where will you fit in?

Use your journal pages to make a list of all the things that scare you about being thin. Now write down a list of all the things you long for in the experience of being thin. You will notice that some of them are very different, yet some are the very same thing.

For example, you might fear the thought of being sexy *and* love the thought of being sexy. Recognizing that ambivalence—seeing how such impulses could cancel each other out—now hand it over to Divine Mind for healing.

Next, write a letter to the new you. Tell her why you fear her, and what makes you nervous about letting her appear. Tell her those things honestly and authentically. But then tell her your deepest truth: that you do love her and hope that she comes. You'll find, in your relationship with her, the key to intimate relationship with anyone: that you're scared, perhaps, but you want to move ahead anyway. That being vulnerable to life in the way love demands is something you have tried to avoid, but you have learned painfully that this does not work. That you're not sure exactly how to do this or how to be with her, but you no longer wish to remain without her. And you apologize for the times you have invited her in and then made her leave.

You are ready to be in the tremulous safety of that which does not always feel safe, for you know now that the citadel of protection you have built around yourself has not protected you from horror and pain. You are willing to let go of the dense energy of false certainty, and embrace at last the light-filled energy of the void. For the void no longer scares you; you realize now that the void is filled with love. The void is where you will find yourself—the place where you become one with the you that is *really* you. And *that* is your miracle: not that you say no to food, but that you say yes to your heart's desire. And saying yes to your heart's desire, you say yes to the possible you.

Miraculously, you are bound by nothing that has occurred before this moment. The fear-mind would be getting hostile by this point, arguing, "Forget it! It's gone on too long! You can't change now!" To which you respond, "Oh yes, I can." For in God there is no past, but only infinite possibilities for a miraculous future. The only way the past can drag you back is if you choose to bring it with you into the present. For the food addict, this takes courage. It takes refusal to believe the false evidence of a worldly mirror. But you are seeing *through* the mirror now, to the real you on the other side of it.

The universe specializes in new beginnings, from the birth of a baby to the appearance of new love. It is the way of nature to begin again, just as it is the way of the fear-mind to stay stuck in the past. You have the ability to change because you are a child of the Divine. Fear would obstruct you, but the hand of God is available to walk you into the dawn of a new day. Do not be concerned about who you were before this moment, for nothing that happened before this instant has power over the will of God. His will is merciful, healing, corrective, and all-powerful. It doesn't matter what the fear-mind says; you will not hear it if you are listening to Him.

Proactively celebrate the arrival of your reborn self. Prepare for her as you would the arrival of a new life, which indeed it is. Every day, take one thing that you know is an aspect of the self now passing—something that perhaps has nothing directly to do with food, yet involves living at a lower energy than that which you are now choosing—and let it go. Perhaps you will get rid of old clutter, or take care of business long overdue. Really, isn't that what weight loss is?

Even when the change *does* have to do with food—perhaps you throw out chemically processed foods, replacing them with fresh fruits and vegetables—the point is not the food specifically. The point is that you are dropping dead energy, lifeless food, lifeless *anything*. You are choosing the aliveness and vitality of whole, natural foods because you are choosing the aliveness and vitality of a new you. You are making the *choice* to be happy. Losing weight is a by-product of choosing to live a happier life.

The thoughts and feelings that make up the new you are coalescing within your mind, your heart, and ultimately the workings of your brain. Just as a nervous system is formed within an embryo, so is a new and different nervous system being formed within you. Your body is at every moment responding to the vibrations of your consciousness, and while some old vibrations might still move through you, you are giving birth to a new body. Cells are constantly dying while new ones are being born—you are literally forming a new physical container.

There is another miraculous aspect of letting go of the past: you can reclaim the love that you denied yourself previously. Every moment you ate food in quality or quantity that was not nourishing, you were denying yourself self-care. But according to *A Course in Miracles,* the love you withheld from yourself in such a moment is held in trust for you until you're ready to receive it.

This means that all the hours of joy you *could* have experienced but did not can be experienced now. They won't come in the same form, but they will reflect the same content. You know that time you went to the beach and were so embarrassed to even be there that you just sat in a café off to the side and told the friends you were with that you didn't really feel like walking along the water? Well, that hour now exists in the ethers of possibility as a joyous walk on the beach you didn't have, could have had, and now *can* have.

The only thing that can stop you now is a failure of imagination. Could the universe really be that merciful? Could the time-space continuum really be that malleable? Could your past really be undone in the future?

You betcha. Unless God is just sorta God, which is always a possibility if you want to think that way. Your material limitations are a reflection of your beliefs, and if you believe that a miracle isn't possible, then there's no reason to expect one.

And expecting one is even more powerful if you're preparing for it. The new you has a different set of attitudes and a different set of habits than the old you; it's helpful to recognize what some of them are so you can more easily align yourself with the energies they represent.

In your journal pages, write down some of the thoughts, feelings, and activities of the new you. Write "The New Me" at the top of a page, and then start making a list. Each line begins: *"I . . . "*

The New Me

- *I . . . go skinny-dipping in the neighborhood pond.*

- *I . . . wear a bathing suit at the beach and do not feel embarrassed.*

- *I . . . walk through a shopping mall and do not feel unhappy.*

- *I . . . get on a scale and feel proud of myself.*

- *I . . . take my clothes off at the doctor's office and do not feel ashamed.*

- *I . . . know what it feels like to be hungry before I eat.*

- *I . . . go to a party and do not feel inadequate.*

- *I . . . enjoy rolling around and playing games on the floor with young children.*

- *I . . . am proud to know that my family is proud of me.*

- *I . . . am more sensitive than I used to be to the suffering of others.*

- *I . . . see food as a gift for which I am grateful to God, which I would never abuse, and which I wish all people to have enough of.*

- *I . . . enjoy my body.*

- *I . . . enjoy taking care of my body.*

- *I . . . give thanks for my body and the joy it brings myself and others.*

Beneath each sentence, embellish further on what you embrace in your new life. Do this by speaking in the first person, as if you were writing in your diary:

> *Today I went to the beach, and enjoyed wearing my new orange cover-up with the gold beads in the front. As I walked across the sand, I enjoyed the feeling of the sun on my skin, the way my body was healthy and toned, and how good it felt to be so light and free.*

Then write these words, or something like them:

> *Praise God; Hallelujah; So be it; Amen;* or *How fabulous is <u>that</u>!!!*

Do not forget to put your writing on the altar when you are done.

You are building new pathways in your brain now, preparing a home for the you who is emerging. But these paths must develop according to your own rhythms and your own choices. The new you isn't the arrival of someone other than you; she is the emergence of whom you have always been but have long kept hidden. It's not that something was *wrong* with you; it's that in the area of weight, something as right with you as with anyone else has been buried by your addictive urge. You were never wrong; you were just wounded. Your need is not to replace some defective self, but to invoke into operation once more the perfect you that is the truth of who you are.

The fear-mind would have you believe none of that: "You are *wrong* because you have this weight problem. You are *wrong* because you haven't dealt with it better." But you are a child of the Divine, and the Divine is not *wrong*. Yes, you've been thrown off the track of your perfection, but your perfection was never destroyed.

In order to manifest your external perfection, you must find once again your internal perfection. But your way might not look like everyone else's. Your essence is not something imposed from without; it is something that emerges organically from within. You give birth to the real you by giving yourself something that perhaps you've never had: the permission to simply *be*.

For whatever reason and in whatever way, the real you has been crouching for years in a corner of your psychic closet. The real you has not shown up in the world as too large; she has shown up as too *small*. And while you have tried desperately to feed her, it is not food—but rather your permission, your approval, and your appreciation—that makes her stand tall and proud. When you feed her emotionally, she will feed you physically. For in giving birth to her, you will become her. And the imposter will fade away.

No wonder you have not had perfect appetites: there is a place where the perfect you has not been given the psychic space to even exist. Now that you see this, you can allow her to emerge. You can stop censoring her. You can stop hiding her. You can stop emotionally aborting your own birth process. And you will find that the real you, once she is allowed to shine, knows exactly what to do, in every area of your life, to cast a radiance and a glow.

You do not need to tell her what to do or how to be; you need only to *allow* her to do and to be what she already is programmed by God to do and be. One thing is sure: like all children of God, she is both perfect and perfectly unique. The last thing you need to do is to tell her how to eat: your miracle lies in allowing *her* to tell *you* how to eat.

In a world of cookie-cutter this and cookie-cutter that, she is anything but cookie-cutter. You're going to lose weight, but you're going to do it *your* way. The real you has a natural wisdom for how best to eat, and a natural wisdom for how best to lose weight. Just know that your pattern might not look like someone else's. Some of us move in circles, and some of us move in a line.

I realized long ago that if I go into my bedroom and tell myself, "Okay, now. Make your bed. Clean up your room. Organize everything," I'm liable to feel completely over-whelmed by the task. But if I tell myself that every time I go into my room, I can make *something* right—make up part of the bed, pick up my shoes and clean up the books in that pile over there, then make up another part of the bed next time I walk in, and so forth—then I will have cleaned up my room in the same amount of time that it might have taken others. I will have just done it in a kind of circular, rather than straight-line, motion. Circles aren't worse than straight lines; they're just a different pattern.

I've discovered the same thing with physical exercise. If I tell myself that I must work out for an hour, then that's sometimes difficult for me—something I'm not likely to do as regularly as I should. But I've discovered that if I have a yoga mat in my office, a set of weights there and another set in my bedroom, an exercise ball in the hallway and an ab machine behind my desk, then I have no problem whatsoever—in fact, I enjoy it—stopping every couple of hours or so and doing about ten minutes of exercise because it feels good! By the end of the day, I've done all the exercise I need.

I realize there are exercise experts who would argue that the continuous motion of a one-hour workout is better, but all I know is that whether it comes to food, exercise, or almost anything else, I have to find my own rhythms and honor them. I tell myself daily that even a short walk or a tiny run is okay. And when I do go to the gym, I don't have to spend an hour there for my time to have been well spent.

My relationship with food is similar. I am not a food addict, so there's no particular food from which I must abstain. Having been a compulsive eater, however, I still have it within me to act that out. A good cake can't sit around my house or I'm likely to eat it. Cookies aren't often in my cupboards because I've learned better. But neither do I deny myself.

The key for me is to let myself have whatever I want, because in so doing, I give myself permission to be who I really am—and who I really am does not *want* to overeat. As long as I allow myself when at a restaurant to order the fruit crumble, I'm likely to eat very little of it. A teaspoon or two might be all I want. But if I don't order it? I'm likely to eat many more calories than that later on in the day, as a reaction to having denied myself.

The real you, like the real me, knows what to do and how to do it. But you must allow yourself to prove that. Limits are good, but they can't be arbitrarily imposed; they must emerge from your own internal wisdom. No one said to me, "Under no circumstances allow cake to sit on your kitchen counter." No, I came up with that one myself. I *choose* not to let cake sit there, out of love for myself and a recognition of my own limitations. If you are an addict and *must* impose certain limits, then know that those limits are a gift to you and receive them as such.

Ultimately, your greatest miracle is this: you'll come to realize that you are fine *exactly as you are*. The real you *wants* healthy food, invigorating exercise, and an active lifestyle. The real you doesn't *want* the damaging effects of unhealthy, chemically processed food and a sedentary existence. The real you knows those things for what they are—a tomb for the person you used to be. You are changed now, and those days are over. They are a thing of the past.

You've had a glimpse in the spiritual mirror and seen the person you were meant to be, who you yearn to be and now choose to be. You are ready to do more than just lose weight. You are ready to rise above, to start again, and to be free.

Reflection and Prayer

Take a deep breath and close your eyes.

See with your inner eye a great fountain of light emerging from your forehead. The water of the fountain is made up of sparkling, liquid light. It is a fountain of true consciousness, spewing love, light, and laughter into the air around you.

Now see these trajectories of light begin to form a shape, and see that the shape they form is the physical body of your Divinely inspired self. Simply *enjoy* this playful, enchanted vision. Do not judge it. Merely see it. You are seeing who you really are.

See the vision grow in detail and solidity, and watch as it begins to look at you. Does she say anything? Receive the love and gratitude that your potential self now pours in your direction. You are celebrating her birth into the world; you are reborn as one. The real you has been hidden for far too long, and she is overjoyed to be emerging now.

Watch what she does and how she moves. See how she expresses herself. Notice how she eats. Spend time with her. Embrace her. *Enjoy her.* And know that she is you.

Dear God,
On this day,
I celebrate my rebirth.
In praise and thanks,
I accept it now.
Help me let go of
the me that was,
and begin again as a better self . . .
a higher self,
a noncompulsive self,
a more joyful self,
a more useful self,
a more peaceful self,
a more loving self,
a more beautiful self,
the self I truly am.
Dear God,
I surrender now,
and give thanks
for what is to be.
Amen

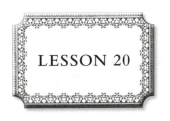

SOUL SURGERY

Imagine yourself once again lying on a white marble slab. The slab may look uncomfortable, but it is not. Where you might expect it to feel hard and cold, it feels instead as though you are falling into a heavenly space of infinite love. It's a soft mattress onto which you can now relax in ways you've never relaxed before, at peace in a way you've never been before. You are not alone, but rather are surrounded by invisible forces. There are angels and people who love you all around.

This image is as real as the chair you are sitting on. And it's not just describing a particular place or experience—it's describing the spiritual reality of your life. The fear-mind audaciously proclaims that *it* has reality on its side: the reality of your body size, the reality of your obsession, the reality of your past failures. But this is where the fear-mind is wrong, for the world it reports to you is merely an illusion. You're awakening from your illusions now, and the material plane as you experience it is beginning to transform.

Every time you encounter anyone, anytime you go anywhere or have any experience at all, you're being invited by the universe to make a choice for the real you. Experience everything now within the light of love, and as you do so, your inner light will shine. It will remind you of your essential knowing, activate your spiritual powers, and bring peace to your internal kingdom.

In the presence of your true self, any word, any choice, any appetite, any energy, any manifestation at all that does not reflect its beauty . . . will simply fall by the wayside. You won't say "No" to bad food choices; you simply won't even consider them. They will no longer call to you.

Once you've aligned yourself with the lightness of your true being, the dense, heavy energies of addiction and compulsion will fall away of their own dead weight. No longer backed by the emotional force of your unprocessed issues, they will have no life force at all. They will drain out of you, their tentacles no longer able to grab on to a system that gives it nothing to grab on to. You have made your decision, and as with any decision made with the force of true love, all contrary energy becomes null and void.

You have begun the process of self-examination that is at the heart of true healing: you have embraced the process; resisted the process; walked away from the process; and still, at moments, opened in a more humble way to the possibility of a miracle. Like every addict, you have both cried out for healing and shut the door to your healing, sometimes in the same breath. But you have made the effort.

You have done this course with love in your heart, and the love you've beckoned is on its way. You have prayed to be released. You have summoned a spiritual healing, and you have opened your heart to receive it. Prepare yourself now for spiritual surgery, the alchemy of Divine Mind once it is given access to your total being.

The Divine Physician will cut away from you all that you do not want. He will remove the weightiness from your heart, and you will know the lightness you yearn for.

Cleanse your heart for this, just as you would cleanse your body before physical surgery. Take several deep breaths, inhaling forgiveness and love and exhaling resentment and fear as best you can. Be willing to open yourself up to a miraculous operation.

Read the following visualization, and then close your eyes to see it. Pray for God's presence, and imagine the Divine Physician coming toward you as you lie on the marble slab. Receive His love, and with your inner eye watch what happens as He places His hands upon you.

Feel the spiritual laser of His love as it enters into you. Allow yourself to feel the emotional issue that is stored in each area of your body, and experience His healing.

People might appear in your mind to apologize to you or to receive your apology; wisdom might come to you that you hadn't previously accessed; direction and guidance for your life might stream into your mind. As this happens, excess flesh begins to fall to the side. On the flesh are imprinted words and issues, hopes and fears, memories and traumas, names and situations . . . words that only you and He can know.

Grief you still carry . . . weaknesses you wish removed . . . problems you've tried to solve without Divine help . . . situations you've tried to steer without Divine guidance . . . goals you've tried to achieve without Divine blessing . . . questions you've tried to answer without praying for wisdom . . . relationships that aren't working . . . relationships for which you haven't been appropriately grateful . . . situations where you know you could do better . . . areas of life where you've been only thinking of yourself . . . the name of a person you have not still forgiven . . . an event you cannot let go of . . . a relationship you cannot stop obsessing about. . . . The places in your mind that have been shut in pain will now relax beneath the hands of the Divine Physician.

Everything that causes you anxiety now falls away. As the weight is removed from your psyche, it is invisibly removed from your body as well. Its energy miraculously turns into wisdom. And the wisdom turns into light.

He has heard every cry you ever cried out to Him, in the depths of your sorrow and despair. He has listened to every prayer you have prayed, and He has watched every effort you have made to be free. Now, with this surgery on your soul, He reprograms your mind and cuts out darkness at its roots. Shame . . . cut away. Judgment and blame . . . cut away. Grief . . . cut away. Fear and burdens . . . cut away. Self-reference . . . cut away. Isolation . . . cut away. Obsession . . . cut away. Anger . . . cut away. Craving . . . cut away.

What remains is your essential self. As you return at last to your Divine reality—to the immaculate, unchangeable love within you—then all thoughts and feelings and appetites are healed. That which does not exist for love no longer exists in you.

In the space of this miraculous process, in the silence of this holy operation, allow yourself to truly experience the movement of the Divine Physician's hand. He removes flesh from your body by removing pain from your heart. This operation is as real as you choose it to be. Your body is healed and your mind is restored. Your miracle has come.

Reflection and Prayer

This entire lesson is a reflection on spiritual reality. Spend as much time with it as you can, and then say the prayer on the next page.

Dear God,
I am ready to heal.
I am ready to let go.
Please take my willingness,
whether weak or strong,
and use it to transform my life.
Enter me, every cell of my being.
Cut out all my dysfunction and disease.
Remove all compulsion and
illumine my heart.
I give to You my darkness,
please fill me with Your light.
Take away what is wrong with me
and leave only what is right.
May I know at last
who I truly am.
Amen

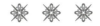

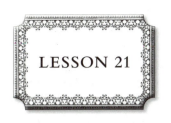

THE BODY BRILLIANT

You are on a journey now that, having started, will never end.

Every time you think God's name, your cells will fall more deeply into Divine alignment. Surrender your body to love, seeing your only function on this earth as being love's hands, feet, words, and actions. Make this like a game you play, imagining that you're living in a holy world. For indeed you are. With every breath you take, you will thrill to breathe in God's spirit. Your entire body will awaken to a new and almost startling aliveness. You live in Him, as He lives in you.

When you look upon your hand, see His hand. When you see through your eyes, imagine you are seeing through His. Several times throughout the day, just stop and imagine that your body is made of light. And light you will be.

Yes, you will lose your weight. Add to this course whatever regimen works for you regarding food and physical exercise, and you've got a winning combination at last. But remember: once you've lost the weight, if you go back to the thought-forms that were stored inappropriately in your flesh to begin with, then it's reasonable to assume that the storage process will resume. You've learned something about yourself from all of this: you do not function well outside the circle of God's love.

All roads, whether filled with darkness or filled with light, circle back in time to the arms of the Divine. Whether through the light at the end of the tunnel or the light that is seen at the moment of death, love will always have the final say. You need not wait for either tunnel or death; you can hear it now. The suffering you've experienced was not love's will to begin with, and you have suffered enough. You know now what to do to stop.

Will you ever be able to eat this or that, whenever you want to? That is not for me to say; those with a far better understanding of your physical circumstances than I would have to advise you about that. Will you ever be able to just forget about serving the dictates of love in everything you do? To that, I can respond quite confidently: *No.* At least not without risk. You've entered into a deep understanding of where your soul most longs to be: held tightly in the arms of God, without the slightest interest in going anywhere else. Outside the encircling warmth of that love, you are not at home, you are agitated on a soul level, and you are likely to do something to act out your agitation. This is not bad news, by the way. It means you're a mystic at heart.

You will never forget what this issue in your life has put you through—and, at the deepest level, you won't really want to. For when you look in the mirror and see only the happy person whose body weight has become a source of pleasure and not pain, you will know that you have seen a miracle. You will know that you have learned a spiritual secret that you could have only found in the depths of your darkness and at the height of your despair.

Even though the tears you cried on the way to your miracle were the tears of someone who wondered at times if life was even worth the pain, you will know in your heart that it was. For ultimately it showed you something about God and about yourself. The person you will be on the other side of this problem, as you continue on your journey far past the station called "Weight Loss," will have a secret smile that only something much more powerful than weight loss itself could have given you. It will not just be your body that is renewed, but also your heart and soul.

And where you will go from there will be a different future than you would have known were you still ravaged and lost in food hell. Having been delivered from that awful place, you will notice those who seek delivery themselves. And with often no more than a gentle smile, but sometimes a more substantial reach, you will be there for others as you have felt the invisible spirit of love reach out for you.

You will be someone who, having received a miraculous healing, can work a miracle in the lives of others. There will be a depth to your words, reflecting the depth of your hard-earned wisdom; a kindness to your spirit, reflecting the celestial touch that reached out to you in the depth of your misery; and a power to your personality that one only encounters in someone who has stared down the devil in his or her own soul. Congratulations. This is not the end; it is your new beginning.

You are not who you were yesterday, you are not who you've been taught to think you are, and you are not your body. You are a spirit who lives eternally in a realm beyond the material world, wearing a physical body like a beautiful suit of clothes. And you don't just know that now. You *truly* know it. It is not just a metaphor; it is truth.

Your spiritual self is not secondary to your material self: It was here before your body was born, and it will live beyond its dying. It is not a symbol; it is who you really are. Beyond your body, there is a body brilliant. And everything you've ever been through, including the horrible paths you have trod through the hell of dysfunctional eating, have ultimately served but one purpose only: to get you here, to this point, to this knowing, and to this peace.

Feel not only the physical; feel the body brilliant. When sitting, feel your body . . . then sense the spiritual body that sits within you. Simply feel its presence; that is all you need do.

Feel not only the physical; feel the body brilliant. When standing, feel your body . . . then sense the spiritual body that stands within you. Simply feel its presence; that is all you need do.

Feel not only the physical; feel the body brilliant. When walking, feel your body . . . then sense the spiritual body that walks within you. Simply feel its presence; that is all you need do.

These are subtle actions, yet they will change your life. For what you feel is what you will feed. The fact that this will diminish your weight is almost incidental. You've given birth to a new sense of self. You are leaving behind a merely material sense of who you are, and identifying instead with the spirit within you. In the spiritual realm, you carry no excess substance, because you are love and love only.

This journey ends a personal nightmare and initiates a more awakened way of walking through life. You have turned to God for help with your weight, and you have felt Him respond; be sure now that you yourself do not abandon the relationship. Weight has been a wounding in your spirit, but it is a wounding that has brought you to your knees—and in that way, it has become a blessing. It has taught you humility, it has brought you to a greater understanding of the awesomeness and mercy of the universe, and it has brought you home to your true self. Now that you've encountered such mysteries, do not allow yourself to forget what they taught you.

You know now that miracles occur naturally in the presence of love, and that your compulsion erupts in the presence of fear. You know that any moment of blocked love is an invitation for fear to enter. You know that fear fuels the ego, activates addiction, and makes inevitable your return to suffering. You know that whenever you choose love, even when your resistance is great, love will always be there to save you from yourself. Remember these things and you will be fine.

That which you have thought of as your greatest burden has, in fact, become your greatest miracle. Any remorse you feel, any regret over pain you've already suffered, will be magically transformed into joy. All the happiness you denied yourself when in the throes of food hell is awaiting you now, having been put in a "Send Later" file while you were overeating. Now you will be able to download all the marvelous, free, and bountiful energies that were deflected by your compulsion. From the pleasure of wearing a cool pair of jeans to the discovery of the value of fresh, organic food; from the fun of dancing to the satisfaction of a healthier lifestyle, you will *enjoy* yourself in a way you have not allowed yourself in quite a while, if ever.

This is a path you'll walk for the rest of your life—not just to manage your food issues, but in order to find and live the truest version of yourself. Your work will be, every day, to vigilantly monitor your thoughts—so you won't *have* to monitor your eating so vigilantly. The lighter your thoughts are, the lighter will be your appetite. As mental and emotional obesity fall to the wayside, then so will their physical counterpart. You will become, throughout all dimensions of your being, your "light-filled" self.

Open your journal once more and ruminate on what this course has been for you . . . what has been difficult, what has been easy, what you feel you've accomplished, and what you feel you will be continuing to work on as you move forward. Write down things you've learned about yourself as you've gone through this course, and what changes you're making as a result of your insights. Notice how your self-perception has changed since realizing that you are so much more than the body of flesh that your physical eyes perceive.

Glance at your altar and think of who you were when you began building it, how much less you understood about yourself, and how much more vulnerable you felt back then to the addictive demons that have so terrorized your life. Regardless of whether you feel that all the demons have yet retreated full-time to their lair in the realms of nothingness, notice how certain you are, somewhere in your mind, that you are not alone in fighting them—and that the battle, in fact, is already won. Know now, and do not forget: there are angels to your left and angels to your right, there are angels in your kitchen and angels always with you. You have called for help, and you have sensed its arrival.

No matter where you are on your journey to light, there is one thing you have realized and should always keep in mind: the darkness is behind you. In fact, the darkness is gone.

Reflection and Prayer

Close your eyes and settle into a relaxed and peaceful place.

Now see in your mind's eye the house you live in. Watch as a band of angels comes to visit. As soon as they arrive, they get busy. First they modify your kitchen. They go to the sink, open the refrigerator, check out the cupboards. You can't tell exactly what they are doing, but you know it's good. They find that secret stash you have and laugh as it disappears in their hands. They are transforming your environment, turning everything into light. They go to your bedroom and open up and organize your closet. They clean out the drawers. They're making everything wonderful.

Then you notice that they go everywhere you go in life, from your home to your car to your workplace to anywhere else. You notice that they are filling up the world. As they look at something, it becomes more beautiful; as they touch an object, it turns into blazing light. And finally, they turn to look at you. By the time they start to pour light upon you, they see in you the light that is already there. They themselves beam more brightly as they look at you. They see your spirit, dressed in a most beautiful suit of clothes: the body brilliant, the body beautiful, the body good.

They bow in honor of the light in you. And there is joy.

Dear God,
Today I walk in gratitude
for the miracles You have worked in me,
for the lightness of my being
and the changes that I feel.
May the chaos of my former self
be only a memory now, dear God.
Thank You, thank You, thank You.
Amen

JOURNAL
PAGES FOR

⁕

A
COURSE
IN
WEIGHT
LOSS

~❧ACKNOWLEDGMENTS❧~

In addition to the inestimable contributions by Oprah Winfrey that were mentioned previously, many others helped bring this book to life as well.

My friend and colleague the compassionate and brilliant Grace Gedeon opened up her heart and her schedule to me, helping me understand things I otherwise would not have understood about the secret hell of addictive eating. She traveled halfway around the world to share her wisdom, and any help this course might give to others could not have happened without the help she gave me. I hope that I have written a book that is worthy of her tremendous contribution.

My friend and literary midwife Andrea Cagan, with her inimitable way of speaking both to my weaknesses and my strengths, helped me greatly as I struggled to put my ideas to paper. As she has been before, she was a great gift to me.

I appreciate Katherine Woodward Thomas for her insight and clarity about her own experience, further deepening my knowledge of the secret life of the overeater.

Thanks to Kathy Freston, my "Inspirer," whom I referred to in Lesson 11. Her book *Quantum Wellness* has helped me and countless others understand the spiritual principles involved in healthy eating.

I thank Reid Tracy for publishing this book, and allowing me the time and space to write it as well as I could.

I deeply appreciate Louise Hay and Jill Kramer for doing their own work so marvelously, enabling me to more effectively do mine.

My thanks to Christy Salinas, Amy Gingery, Jacqui Clark, Jeannie Liberati, and Margarete Nielsen for their excellent and gracious approach to the publishing process.

And to Shannon Littrell, my gratitude is deep for the inspiring and always encouraging support. Some people are like literary angels, and you are one.

This book has been a work of love, created and tended to by many loving hands. To all those above, I am deeply grateful.

ABOUT
THE AUTHOR

Marianne Williamson is an internationally acclaimed lecturer and the best-selling author of *A Return to Love, Healing the Soul of America, A Woman's Worth, Illuminata, Everyday Grace, The Gift of Change,* and *The Age of Miracles,* among other works. Williamson has done extensive charitable organizing throughout the country in service to people with life-challenging illnesses (she founded Project Angel Food in Los Angeles). She also founded the grassroots campaign to establish a U.S. Department of Peace.

To learn more about Williamson's work, and to join her e-mail list for notices regarding her lectures and events, visit her Website: **www.marianne.com**.

HAY HOUSE TITLES OF RELATED INTEREST

YOU CAN HEAL YOUR LIFE, the movie,
starring Louise L. Hay & Friends
(available as a 1-DVD program and an expanded 2-DVD set)
Watch the trailer at: **www.LouiseHayMovie.com**

THE SHIFT, the movie,
starring Dr. Wayne W. Dyer
(available as a 1-DVD program and an expanded 2-DVD set)
Watch the trailer at: **www.DyerMovie.com**

*THE ART OF EXTREME SELF-CARE: Transform Your Life
One Month at a Time,* by Cheryl Richardson

*LOSING YOUR POUNDS OF PAIN: Breaking the Link
Between Abuse, Stress, and Overeating,* by Doreen Virtue

*THE SPARK: The 28-Day Breakthrough Plan for Losing Weight,
Getting Fit, and Transforming Your Life,* by Chris Downie

*UNLOCK THE SECRET MESSAGES OF YOUR BODY! A 28-Day Jump-
Start Program for Radiant Health and Glorious Vitality,* by Denise Linn

YOU CAN HEAL YOUR LIFE, by Louise L. Hay

All of the above are available at your local bookstore,
or may be ordered by contacting Hay House (see next page).

We hope you enjoyed this Hay House book.
If you would like to receive a free catalogue featuring additional
Hay House books and products, or if you would like information
about the Hay Foundation, please contact:

Hay House UK Ltd
292B Kensal Road • London W10 5BE
Tel: (44) 20 8962 1230; Fax: (44) 20 8962 1239
www.hayhouse.co.uk

***

Published and distributed in the United States of America by:
Hay House, Inc. • PO Box 5100 • Carlsbad, CA 92018-5100
Tel: (1) 760 431 7695 or (1) 800 654 5126;
Fax: (1) 760 431 6948 or (1) 800 650 5115
www.hayhouse.com

***

Published and distributed in Australia by:
Hay House Australia Ltd • 18/36 Ralph Street • Alexandria, NSW 2015
Tel: (61) 2 9669 4299, Fax: (61) 2 9669 4144
www.hayhouse.com.au

***

Published and distributed in the Republic of South Africa by:
Hay House SA (Pty) Ltd • PO Box 990 • Witkoppen 2068
Tel/Fax: (27) 11 467 8904
www.hayhouse.co.za

***

Published and distributed in India by:
Hay House Publishers India • Muskaan Complex • Plot No.3
B-2• Vasant Kunj • New Delhi - 110 070
Tel: (91) 11 41761620; Fax: (91) 11 41761630
www.hayhouse.co.in

***

Distributed in Canada by:
Raincoast • 9050 Shaughnessy St • Vancouver, BC V6P 6E5
Tel: (1) 604 323 7100
Fax: (1) 604 323 2600

***

Sign up via the Hay House UK website to receive the Hay House
online newsletter and stay informed about what's going on with your
favourite authors. You'll receive bimonthly announcements
about discounts and offers, special events, product highlights,
free excerpts, giveaways, and more!
www.hayhouse.co.uk

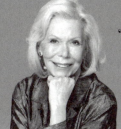
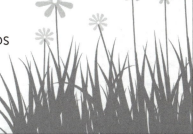

JOIN THE HAY HOUSE FAMILY

As the leading self-help, mind, body and spirit publisher in the UK, we'd like to welcome you to our family so that you can enjoy all the benefits our website has to offer.

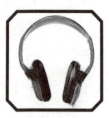 **EXTRACTS** from a selection of your favourite author titles

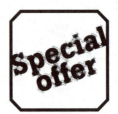 **COMPETITIONS, PRIZES & SPECIAL OFFERS** Win extracts, money off, downloads and so much more

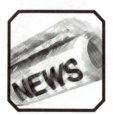 **LISTEN** to a range of radio interviews and our latest audio publications

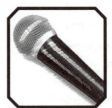 **CELEBRATE YOUR BIRTHDAY** An inspiring gift will be sent your way

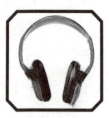 **LATEST NEWS** Keep up with the latest news from and about our authors

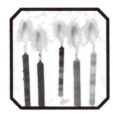 **ATTEND OUR AUTHOR EVENTS** Be the first to hear about our author events

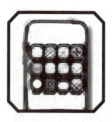 **iPHONE APPS** Download your favourite app for your iPhone

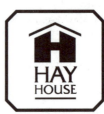 **HAY HOUSE INFORMATION** Ask us anything, all enquiries answered

join us online at **www.hayhouse.co.uk**

292B Kensal Road, London W10 5BE
T: 020 8962 1230 E: info@hayhouse.co.uk